# Counseling in Communication Disorders

## A Wellness Perspective

*Second Edition*

S0-AYW-799

# Counseling in Communication Disorders

## A Wellness Perspective

*Second Edition*

**Audrey L. Holland, PhD**
**Ryan L. Nelson, PhD**

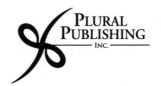

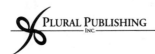

PLURAL PUBLISHING
INC.

5521 Ruffin Road
San Diego, CA 92123

e-mail: info@pluralpublishing.com
Website: http://www.pluralpublishing.com

Copyright © by Plural Publishing, Inc. 2014

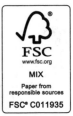

Typeset in 11/13 Garamond by Flanagan's Publishing Services, Inc.
Printed in the United States of America by McNaughton & Gunn, Inc.

Library of Congress Cataloging-in-Publication Data

Holland, Audrey L., author.
  Counseling in communication disorders : a wellness perspective /
Audrey L. Holland, Ryan L. Nelson. — Second edition.
      p. ; cm.
  Includes bibliographical references and index.
  ISBN-13: 978-1-59756-536-3 (alk. paper)
  ISBN-10: 1-59756-536-9 (alk. paper)
  I. Nelson, Ryan L., author. II. Title.
  [DNLM: 1. Communication Disorders—psychology. 2. Counseling—methods. 3. Family Relations. WL 340.2]
  RC428.8
  616.85'506—dc23
                                        2013028584

# CONTENTS

# FOREWORD

"No pessimist ever discovered the secret of the
stars or sailed an uncharted land, or opened a new
doorway for the human spirit."

Helen Keller 1890–1968

*H*elen Keller's words about optimism, growth, and discovery, which I selected for the foreword to the first edition of this book, fit the second edition perfectly as well. In this edition, Audrey Holland and her new coauthor, Ryan Nelson, have maintained Holland's original emphasis on adopting a positive theoretical and philosophical perspective on counseling individuals with communication disorders. This starts with identifying what is right with people who have communication disorders as a means to help them and their families mobilize their strengths to deal with the adversities that have befallen them as a result of an unexpected event. By making positive psychology the "theoretical heart" of this book, Holland and Nelson show clinicians (in training or on the firing line) how to help their students, clients, patients, and families see their glasses as half full rather than half empty.

Positive psychology has evolved, however, since 2006–2007 when the first edition was written. In this edition, Audrey and Ryan draw on the newer work to extend their theoretical framework in ways that parallel Barbara Fredrickson's broaden-and-build theory as discussed in the text. They take the gutsy step from their still-important commitment to providing a pathway to personal happiness to the more encompassing and far-reaching goal of helping individuals to flourish. Expanding on the initial core importance of positive affect, they have stretched the model toward a vision of positive social flourishing. They show how clinicians can augment their central work on improving speech, language, and audition by giving equal footing to engagement, relationship with others, meaning, and accomplishment. They promote these factors as essential to flourishing, both individually and societally.

All of these concepts fit snugly with a fundamental view of human communication as central to personal growth and a key to interpersonal interaction. Although the focus remains on positive affect among the central characters, Audrey and Ryan have built on working with the supporting cast as well and within the communicative systems and networks in which individuals with communication disorders are situated. This includes broadening childhood concerns to focus more explicitly on family involvement in clinical work by speech-language pathologists and audiologists engaged in early intervention, as well as focusing more attention on the school environment (here building on one of Ryan's strengths) for children in their school-age years. Finally, they have broadened the organizational themes beyond wellness, crisis and catastrophe, narrative, and shared expertise, to include the theme of change. Change, in fact, is the meta-goal, the bread and butter, of all clinical efforts.

In my foreword to the previous edition of this work, I stressed my admiration for Audrey's contributions over the years to understanding the essentially social role of language and how that is buffeted about by communication problems. Her view of communication as something authentic, meaningful, and (potentially) fun has set a course for me in much of my research and practice. Now I find that Ryan Nelson clearly shares her values. Although he is new to this edition and to me (and not related), Audrey calls him my descendent. I am honored to learn that he has expressed this as well. Ryan's passion and respect for children and their families, and the importance of context and self-image, are manifest in this book's child chapters, and if that makes him my descendant, I am happy to claim him.

Along with Audrey and Ryan, I recognize the pervasive need for communication specialists to incorporate counseling principles into their practice. Thus, I am extremely pleased to be able to offer this foreword to an updated and expanded version of their unconventional and practical approach to accomplishing that goal.

Nickola Wolf Nelson
Charles Van Riper Professor
Department of Speech Pathology
    and Audiology
Western Michigan University
Kalamazoo, MI

# PREFACE

𝒯his book comes from our hearts. It is not a scientific treatise on counseling; rather, it describes a counseling attitude and explores how speech-language pathologists and audiologists can enrich their clinical practice using specific skills and techniques that incorporate that attitude.

The book also has a strong theoretical orientation in positive psychology and wellness. This means that it basically abandons our profession's long history of building our counseling on principles intended for the treatment of individuals with recognized psychopathology. Instead we build on principles that essentially emphasize what is right with people. We believe strongly that across the lifespan, people (and their families) who incur communication disorders have a far greater likelihood of being recipients of unfortunate things that happen to many of us as we bumble along in the essentially big normal space in the middle of the Gaussian distribution, instead of clustering around its lower edges. Essentially this has made us wonder why our profession's counseling foundation is based on (perfectly good but inappropriate) counseling principles that are intended for helping people with "problems."

Although "on-the-firing line" professionals who pick up this book might be able to sneak around its child chapters if they work with adults, or its adult chapters if infants and school-age children are the focus, this is tricky business, and students (bless you) cannot circumvent any of them. In fact, all the chapters relate to each other and are intertwined. We believe that a thorough reading of the whole book and the interplay among its various parts is a way to get the most out of it. Our hope is that as you read each of the first three chapters, you will experience the same synergistic feeling we did as we attempted to explain the foundations of positive psychology and counseling. The next four chapters illustrate and apply these principles across the lifespan and in a variety of traditional settings. Chapter 8 presents an additional model for helping clients and families benefit from the principles of wellness detailed in earlier chapters. A framework for conducting workshops specifically teaching resilience and optimism is described with a number of practical examples and activities. We close the book with a gift from Stan Goldberg: His Chapter 9 considers the communication counseling issues associated with death and dying through the attitude of dignity and reverence it deserves.

We have loved cooperating on the writing of this new edition. Audrey learned a tremendous amount from Ryan about toddlers and school-age children, and issues faced by speech-language pathologists and audiologists in school settings. In turn, Audrey's expertise with adults and life coaching and counseling greatly enhanced Ryan's understanding. We hardly ever got even slightly annoyed with each other during our long-distance cooperative efforts. So we guess this is what happens when two people who have caught the positive psychology bug work on a project such as this. We positively enjoyed the experience and hope that you do, too.

Namasté ~

Audrey Holland, Tucson, AZ
Ryan Nelson, Lafayette, LA

# ACKNOWLEDGMENTS

**From Audrey:** Believing strongly in the importance of expressions of gratitude, I remain indebted to the endless list I included in my solo edition of this book, and with the same enthusiasm for their influence on my thinking. It pervades the book. For example, I have no idea how many times we have referenced M.E.P. Seligman. What is important here is to recognize those people who have joined that list.

First of all, there is the counseling class that I was privileged to teach right after the first edition of this book became available. One of my students was Ryan, who drove in every week from his duties as an Assistant Professor at the University of Texas El Paso (hardly an easy commute to Tucson). He absolutely enriched and enlivened the class, particularly because he understood far better than I, the adult language person, the unique problems and perspectives of children, parents, and particularly school clinicians. He also brought the class to life and gave me an education I knew I needed. I would probably have let the first edition die without his new perspectives. So I hereby acknowledge my new co-author.

I still need to acknowledge my family, however. Katie, Mike, and their children Tom and Anne, and Ben's son Adrian, infuse my life with joy. Without that, I would be lost. In addition, I acknowledge Richard Parker and Vincent (my pussycats). It is said that dogs have masters and that cats have staff. I serve with them and Pacha Mama (the name I have given a cat that strayed into my backyard) gratitude.

**From Ryan:** Thank you Audrey for letting me work with you! One cannot understand the field of communicative disorders without becoming aware of Audrey's consistently avant-garde influence and contributions. She has shaped this field in ways few others have or ever will.

I first met Audrey the afternoon my wife and I experienced a devastating personal loss. She was in town doing a workshop and yet so naturally and graciously transformed into a friend, helping a couple she had just met grieve by providing a shoulder of comfort and support. Her impact on my life was profound then and remains so today. She has welcomed me into her world, and I am honored that she has invited me to co-author this edition of her book. Her wisdom, expertise, and guidance on this project have enhanced my life immensely.

I must also acknowledge my wonderful friend and former department chair (and former student of Audrey), Anthony P. Salvatore. He encouraged me and allowed my new assistant professor schedule to have the flexibility to pursue my interests in positive psychology and counseling.

There is a tie that binds us to our home and I must acknowledge those who keep me safely and joyfully tethered. To my wife, Tammie, and my three sons (P, B, & J), thank you for loving support and seemingly endless patience. To my astoundingly supportive parents, Bobby and Mikey (both life-long educators), who would never admit their shock of seeing my name on a book! Finally, to Jack Damico for the continued introduction to the life of the mind and the sound advice, "One does not pass up an opportunity to associate with Audrey Holland!"

**From both authors:** There are two people who have shown us incredible generosity. Stan Goldberg knows more than perhaps any other speech-language pathologist about the role of communication counselors in helping people as they move along in the dying process. We are honored that he has once again agreed to author the book's last chapter, and once again, it comes as his gift to us. Thank you, dear friend. Furthermore, the famed rodeo photographer, Louise Serpa, was a friend and role model to Audrey in the last years of her life. As a generous gift, Louise permitted me to use the cover photograph, and she proudly displayed the book in her living room until her death over a year ago. It so completely captures what we are trying to accomplish in this book that the cover had to remain unchanged. Wherever her spirit is, we know that this really pleases her. Thank you, dear friend.

# CONTRIBUTORS

**Stan Goldberg, PhD**
Professor Emeritus Communicative Disorders
San Francisco State University
San Francisco, CA
*Chapter 9*

**Audrey L. Holland, PhD**
Regents' Professor Emerita
University of Arizona
Tucson, AZ

**Ryan L. Nelson, PhD**
Doris B. Hawthorne-BORSF Endowed Professor I
University of Louisiana
Lafayette, LA

# Chapter 1

# COUNSELING IN CLINICAL PRACTICE: OVERVIEW

## Introduction

Speech-language pathologists and audiologists (SLP-As) bring expertise in specific clinical areas to the evaluation and management of communication disorders. Both students and practicing clinicians need to develop counseling skills if they are to serve clients and their families effectively. Counseling is necessary to support decisions and behaviors that optimize quality of life. Knowledge of effective counseling techniques supplements the professional's knowledge about communication disorders and his or her skills in managing these disorders. Finally, appropriate counseling greatly increases the opportunity for an optimal outcome for clients, whether this involves resolving a specific disorder or maximizing quality of life by means of coping and adjustment techniques.

The role of speech-language-hearing professionals is usually complex. Children with severe hearing losses or cerebral palsy, along with their families, face lifelong struggles. Complex problems arise at the other end of the age spectrum as well: Adults who acquire aphasia or dementia, for example, must learn to deal with profoundly changed lives. Our treatment goals for individuals with communication disorders are certainly to minimize the disorder's effects, but counseling also can help involved persons to live productively and successfully with the communication problems, or despite them, or around them.

Effective counseling principles are both learnable and fairly general: The techniques and skills are similar for helping a family with a new baby who has a cleft palate or a hearing deficit and for supporting an adult client with poststroke aphasia, and his family, who face the realities of living with impaired communication. The disorder-specific facts differ, of course, and require disorder-specific understanding of them as well. According to the American Speech-Language-Hearing Association's (ASHA) Scope of Practice statements for speech-language pathology (2007) and for audiology (2004), counseling is an integral part of clinical responsibility for both families and children with speech, language, and hearing disorders, and for adults who have acquired such disorders. Counseling is the basic tool we have to help our clients achieve their lifelong goals. SLP-As often feel uncomfortable about the counseling role, however, and consequently are reluctant to undertake it.

A number of reasons may underlie this reluctance. Perhaps a lack of explicit training in counseling explains it. During our professional education, we are given a wealth of information about the potential problems confronting individuals and families with communication disorders but are taught very little about how the counseling process can be used to help resolve them. Indeed, the ASHA provides no curriculum requirements for SLPs. In their case, it is likely to be tagged onto the end of disorder-specific courses, rather than presented in its own right as a skill to be learned through coursework and practice. The curriculum for AuDs is more enlightened: a counseling course is required.

Counseling for individuals with communication problems has been strongly influenced in the past by traditional concepts derived for counseling individuals with psychological problems. Basic information concerning Freudian defense mechanisms, and the client-centered approaches pioneered by Carl Rogers (1995), have been particularly influential in our field. We suspect that another factor contributing to the reluctance of SLPs to assume a counseling role is that we recognize the implicit mismatch between the forms of counseling originally developed for individuals with disorders such as anxiety or depression and problems faced by individuals who stutter, or for a family with financial problems stemming from the breadwinner's Parkinson disease or incapacitation following a motor vehicle accident.

People who are in need of communication counseling are likely to have been coping with their lives fairly normally before the onset of the communication disorder. This is not to say that individuals with psychological or behavioral problems are immune to communication problems, but a majority of the people for whom SLP-As provide counseling or coaching probably react to the world in ways that are not pathologic. The abnormal models of counseling do not fit very well; they are difficult to apply in clinical practice, even after we have taken a course or two in abnormal psychology. Most communication problems have unique, significant, and reverberating effects on families, who are likely to be as unprepared for them as those who actually incur the problems. Our discipline's reliance on abnormal psychology has seldom been questioned or examined, although it may explain at least partially why many practitioners feel uneasy with their counseling roles.

In this book, counseling for communication disorders has a different theoretical perspective. This approach requires essentially abandoning a treatment model based on what is *wrong* with people who have such disorders. Instead, the emphasis is on what is *right* with them, and how they can mobilize their strengths to deal with the adversities that have befallen them as the result of an unexpected event that threatens one of the most basic human characteristics—the ability to communicate. Thus, the counseling process starts with the assumption that the cup is half full, not half empty. Before onset or recognition of a communication disorder, the affected person and his or her family—whether an adult client who has experienced a stroke with resultant aphasia or the parent of a newborn infant who has been found to be at risk for such a disorder, for example—probably already have been coping reasonably well with life stresses. How do we as counselors capitalize on, and build on, the positive?

## Themes of Interest

Five themes that focus on how to help individuals with communication disorders to develop optimism and resilience constitute a framework for this book. These themes are described next, in no implied hierarchy; all are equally important.

### Theme 1: Wellness and Positive Psychology

Much of the content of this book is based on a conviction that appropriate models and approaches for communication counseling should be grounded in what we know about normality and wellness rather than in what we know about illness and psychopathology. The recent explosion of information about and interest in positive psychology provides the best example, particularly as it is illuminated by the work of M. E. P. Seligman and his colleagues. Here is just a sampling of relevant books on positive psychology published since 2002, following the publication of Seligman's *Authentic Happiness*, which was published then. Some of these important books include: Ben-Shahar, 2010; Diener and Biswas-Diener, 2008; Fredrickson, 2009; Haidt, 2006; Peterson, 2006; Reivich and Shatté, 2002; and Seligman's most recent book (2011), which significantly increases the worldview of the movement. More detailed exploration is central to Chapter 2 of this book.

The first theme of this book is its reliance on the principles and tenets of *positive psychology*, focusing on mental health and well-being and how to achieve and maintain them. Positive psychology is oriented away from illness and toward wellness, both for understanding what it means to live positively and for providing ways to increase authentic happiness in one's own life and to promote a healthier society in general. This book links those principles to counseling individuals and families who experience and live with communication disorders.

One of the most appealing aspects of focusing on wellness and positive psychology as a counseling model in communication disorders is that it fits squarely with the facet of counseling with which SLP-As are most comfortable: providing information. We are skilled educators and good providers of information. Training in speech-language pathology and audiology produces good teachers, whether we are teaching children to move a lateral lisp into a more acceptable /s/ production, or reestablishing semantic skills in aphasic adults, or teaching effective hearing aid use. Counseling is a change process, as are many of the other techniques used by SLP-As. To the extent that our counseling can capitalize on our teaching skills, we can become comfortable with a counseling role.

A core feature of positive psychology is its development of explicit ways to increase resilience and optimism. These two attributes are particularly critical for learning to cope with the many disasters or catastrophes that occur in the process of simply living life. Basic principles of positive psychology are covered in Chapter 2, and a number of its experimentally validated exercises are presented there. Other exercises that have been adapted specifically for communication counseling are scattered throughout the book.

## Theme 2: Living the Catastrophe, Dealing with Crisis

In this book, the words "catastrophe" and "catastrophic" generally are used in the conventional sense of *disaster* and *disastrous*. They imply the kinds of wrenching problems that result from the spectrum of communication disorders ranging from developmental disorders discovered in infancy to the dementias that occur late in life. But *catastrophe* is also used in this book in the sense that Jon Kabat-Zinn used it in his book on stress reduction and meditation, *Full Catastrophe Living* (anniversary edition, 2005). Kabat-Zinn borrowed his title in part from Kazantzakis' *Zorba the Greek* (1996). In the film adaptation of Kazantzakis' book, Zorba responds to the question of whether he was ever married: "Of course I've been married. Wife, house, kids, everything . . . the full catastrophe!" Kabat-Zinn interpreted Zorba's remark as a basic appreciation of the roller-coaster nature of being alive. This usage of the word *catastrophe* embodies the spirit of accepting change and knowing that, in Kabat-Zinn's words:

> . . . it is not a disaster to be alive just because we feel fear and we suffer . . . [to understand] that there is joy as well as suffering, hope as well as despair, calm as well as agitation, love as well as hatred, health as well as illness . . . (p. 5)

The "full catastrophe" for most people involves good *and* bad, easy *and* hard, periods of happiness *and* periods of pain. In fact, someone who manages to avoid the negatives may be perceived in some way as diminished (and perhaps likely to be rather boring!). Although the issues we deal with in our communication counseling gravitate toward the negative pole, it is crucial to remember that the opposite, the positive, also is there. Good counselors respect and honor not only their clients and their problems but also the "full catastrophe" of the human condition.

Crisis models may be useful for clinicians who deal with the full catastrophe of parents experiencing that their child has Down syndrome, or that aphasia has resulted from the stroke one's husband has incurred. Before most people can accept the bad, they have to acknowledge it and come to peace with it. Crisis models, developed by Elisabeth Kübler-Ross for dealing with grief, death, and dying (1969), have been useful with many chronic health issues as well. Although her model has significant shortcomings, as adapted by Webster and Newhoff (1981) for our professions it can be useful for elucidating the process whereby individuals can learn to deal with catastrophic events.

Four stages are postulated to occur as individuals progress toward healthy resolution. These stages are called various names by various authors. In this book, Webster and Newhoff's terms are used. These are, in order, shock, realization, retreat, and acknowledgment. Certainly, not all individuals go through all stages in an orderly fashion, and not all individuals actually reach satisfactory acknowledgment. In fact, Goldberg (2006) commented that in his extensive experience as a hospice counselor, he has never observed an individual who followed precisely these stages of grief. Nevertheless, these stages should be kept in mind by SLP-As for their counseling work with parents, spouses, and persons who have experienced sudden catastrophic illnesses.

Immediately after a catastrophe, neither the family nor the person who has experienced it is in a particularly good position to take advantage of information concerning the problem offered then. Nevertheless, almost without exception, experienced clinicians routinely provide such information. Frequently, however, SLPs whose work focuses on chronic aphasia hear comments from clients and their families that "things were not explained" and that they had no idea what to expect. In such instances, the shock of the stroke may compromise the ability of the affected person and family members to absorb new information in the earliest stages of recovery. This limitation does not mean that clinicians should stop providing information in the initial aftermath of a potentially disabling event. But we should not be surprised when affected individuals and families fail to comprehend all of the early information they receive, and we should be prepared to repeat it, perhaps frequently.

Of greater importance, this initial failure to comprehend or retain relevant information means that the first of Webster's (1977) counseling functions—listening—should be primary. Webster points out that listening to what people wish to share and to their fears about the future, and simply holding hands and being present, are what matters at this time. It also is valuable to provide information that is more permanent than the spoken word. Pamphlets, videotapes, and contact information sheets and the like will be useful later, when the realization stage is reached. Once the client and family members realize what this problem may actually entail, written information and relevant telephone numbers can be used productively.

Retreat is likely to be the least universal of these four crisis stages, at least for the types of problems encountered by SLP-As; however, retreat can manifest as denial that a problem actually exists or that the disorder will have a major impact in the long run. For example, Dora, the spouse of a man who has recently suffered a major stroke, comments, "Ralph may have global aphasia, but you don't know his will. He'll be back to work at his old job in 6 months, mark my words." As counselors, we must be aware of the delicate nature of such denial, as well as of the need to deal with denial when it occurs.

It is not uncommon for clinics to have spouses rate communication of their communication-impaired partner using the Communication Effectiveness Index (CETI) (Lomas, Pickard, Bester, Elbard, Findlayson, & Zoghabib, 1989). A frequent outcome is that early in the rehab process, spouses rate their partners as substantially higher than on CETIs taken later in the recovery process. After families have lived with a disorder for a longer period of time, problems often become more apparent. When Dora realizes Ralph is not back at work yet, and that their future may be very different from the one she has envisioned, counseling offers the mechanism for her reassessment.

Acknowledgment of the problem is not a synonym for giving up. Acknowledgment is recognizing the reality of the individual's condition, making room for the changes, and moving on with life. Ram Dass (2000, p. 185), who completed his book *Still Here* after experiencing a stroke that resulted in aphasia and hemiplegia, eloquently described the good that resulted from acknowledging his deficit. He comments:

> The stroke was like a samurai sword, cutting apart the two halves of my life. It was a demarcation between the two stages. In a way, it's been like having two incarnations in one; this is me that was "him" . . . Seeing it that way saves me from the suffering of making comparisons, of thinking about the things I used to do but can't do anymore because of the paralysis in my hand. In the "past incarnation" I had an MG with a stick shift, I had golf clubs, I had a cello. Now I don't have any use for those things! New incarnation!

## Theme 3: Change

Implicit in the above is that, as people live into their "full catastrophes" and move through their crises, differing counseling needs may appear, as well as different strategies for clinical management of problems that have evolved. Change is a reality of life, but this is a profession that counts on our knowing how to make it happen. Change is often assumed to be a matter of applying some behavioral techniques we learned in psychology class to the communication problems we learned about in excruciating detail in graduate school. But change is hard, and it demands some attention in its own right.

Consider 5-year-old Alan with a relatively clear-cut phonological problem involving his use of /s/. Alan began talking at around 2 years of age, and the /s/ sound he started out with is the one he continues to use. None of us can dare to estimate how much practice he has had with it, but all of us can see the difficulty of expecting him to change it in a semester's worth of clinical time. *That* we would like to get him to change is one thing; *how* to accomplish it is another. The techniques for effecting this are within our counseling purview (and involve his parents and Alan, of course).

Change issues are not unique to children. The issues become accentuated with communication disorders in aging. Lifestyles, attitudes, behaviors that increase the probability of another stroke, and role reversals all involve changes. Here is a pertinent clinical example: An aging investment banker who has recently suffered an aphasia-producing stroke must learn to trust the clinician sitting across from him as she instructs him on word finding, that is, following the advice of a clinician likely to be nearer his daughter's age than his own. The task, the situation and its history, and the age gap all potentially require some element of change if they are to be managed well. We consider change and how to effect it more directly in Chapter 3, but change is a pervasive theme throughout our clinical work and shows up in other chapters as well. Change, however, serves as a good introduction to our next theme.

## Theme 4: Who Are the Experts?

The social model of disability has been growing in strength and influence over the past 30 years. It has significant implications for the practice of speech-language pathology and audiology. Perhaps its greatest significance relates to our profession's counseling functions. Briefly put, the social model makes it clear that disability itself is not a problem of disabled persons alone; it also is a substantial result of living in disabling societies. Furthermore, disability is perhaps not a tragedy but a fact of life (part of the whole catastrophe, as it were). Finally, the problems faced by people with disabilities are broad social ones, requiring similarly broad social solutions and sweeping attitudinal change on the part of the nondisabled, including the professionals who work with them.

The disability movement (Barnes, Mercer, & Shakespeare, 1999; Oliver, 1996) embodies those social concerns and has had a significant impact on the development of the International Classification of Functioning and Disability (ICF) (World Health Organization, 2001). Although full discussion of the ICF is beyond the scope of this book, it is a topic with which all SLP-As must become familiar. One important implication for counseling is that the social model of disability insists that societies rethink the question of expertise in relation to any disabling condition. It asks the question, "Who is the expert?" This question has powerful ramifications for counseling. People with disabilities have strongly challenged the traditional assumption that *professional* is synonymous with *expert*. In this book, we challenge that assumption as well.

The initial approach to counseling should recognize that as SLP-As, we have an undeniable expertise consisting of our technical knowledge and our ability to compile the resources that might be available to our clients. But does this expertise ensure that we are the experts? In fact, at least one and possibly two or three other experts are involved. One of these other experts is the person who lives *in* the disorder. (This is particularly relevant for adolescents and adults who have incurred their disorders after they have achieved some autonomy.) The final experts are those who live *with* the disorder. This means families and significant others. In much the same way in which meaning in conversation is co-constructed by a speaker and a listener, counseling is co-constructed by these experts—that is, the disabled person, those whose lives are connected to the disabled person, and the counselor.

This expanded concept of "expert" became apparent to Audrey even before the advent of the social model of disability. As a beginning clinician, I often found myself smugly amused when parents would comment about their child, "He never acts like this at home." "Hmm," I would think, "it's amazing what sort of blinders parents wear, particularly if experts aren't around." Then I had children. The first time I heard myself utter, "He isn't like this at home," I recognized my professional limitations as the expert. I learned that as clinicians, we could claim only one of the two or three places at the experts' table. Ryan's experiences in fatherhood led him to the same conclusion.

## Theme 5: The Importance of Stories

The fifth theme of this book involves narrative as it relates to problem solving and counseling. Telling one's own story is part of the healing process that precedes the development of resilience and optimism. It is crucial. Illness narratives contain a lot of the narrator's power; see the writings of Coles (1989), Frank (1995), and Kleinman (1988) for excellent examples of the genre of illness narrative. Hinckley (2006) and Shadden, Hagstrom, and Koski (2008) have addressed this topic in relation to stories written by persons with aphasia and other neurogenic communication disorders and their families. In his novel *Still Life with Woodpecker* (1980), Tom Robbins notes that we "all star in our own movie."

This is a profound notion.[1] We learn from ourselves as we hear ourselves tell our own stories. We also learn when we listen to each other's stories (in effect, when we "go to" each other's movies) and derive important lessons and role models from them. When interviewer Charlie Rose recently asked U2's Bono to tell his story, the truly remarkable musician and humanitarian commented that "Everybody's story is valuable . . . mine is not more important than everyone else's."

A sage aphasic client pointed out that one of the most healing aspects of his aphasia group was the frequent ritual of each group member telling the story of his or her stroke and the progress that person has made since its onset. These stories never lost their centrality, and each new member was always welcomed into the group with telling and sharing the stories of the veteran group members, as well as the story of the new member. When Holland, Cherney, and Halper (2010) asked a fairly large sample of aphasic individuals to develop monologues that they subsequently learned to produce, the clear topic of choice was the story of their aphasia. In most cases their narratives included comments reminding their listeners that they were the same person they were before the stroke, and that they continued to get better, however long ago their stroke occurred.

Accordingly, stories about real people with real communication problems appear frequently throughout this book. These stories are positive but usually not heroic. They are simply everyday instances of getting along with life, of moving on. They reflect the importance of positive attitudes and behaviors, and they serve to remind us of the importance of finding and using such stories and role models in counseling.

### Summary of Themes

Wellness and positive psychology, the full catastrophe and crisis, change, shared expertise, and narrative, are essential elements of the counseling approach developed in this book. These elements

---

[1]But as Chodron (2001) points out, "It is possible to move through the drama of our lives without believing so earnestly in the character we play." This serves as a reminder of our role in the big scheme of things, and of our need for perspective. This is important, too.

form the basis for the concepts, techniques, skills, and exercises presented throughout the text as tools to increase the effectiveness of SLP-As in counseling clients and families across the spectrum of communication disorders. First, however, a number of definitions need to be clarified to permit their use as a kind of shorthand in the rest of this book. Finally, a few other topics, such as the role of group and individual counseling, are dealt with briefly in this overview.

## Definitions

### What Is Counseling in Communication Disorders?

Counseling is, above all, a listening process. The first task of this process involves *trying to understand how the world looks to clients*. This requires careful self-examination of the SLP-A's personal, subjective worldview, and then systematically taking the steps necessary to remove personal biases that would compromise the listening process. Once unbiased listening has been learned and practiced, we can apply it in our counseling for clients whose worldview, cultural beliefs, and personal principles may differ significantly from our own. The ability to see how the world looks to our clients provides the context for understanding and acceptance that makes clients comfortable enough to express their feelings, concerns, anxieties, and so forth. The second task of counseling is to *encourage their expression*. The clinical atmosphere for counseling must ensure that a client feels safe, as well as cherished and respected. The third task in the counseling process is *advising*, that is, providing the information that people need to help them understand what is happening to them, as well as showing them how to get on with their lives and live in a realistic fashion, with both optimism and resilience. Then comes the last task of counseling and the most difficult step: *helping individuals to translate information into satisfying and successful actions*. (Note that in this paragraph, the themes of wellness, narrative, and change have already come up.)

The goal of the counseling process is to help individuals and families to live as successfully as they possibly can, despite the intrusion of events such as a motor vehicle accident that results in a child's traumatic brain injury, a stroke that occurs just as retirement is nearing, a dawning awareness of an infant's developmental disability, or any of a score of other catastrophic events that result in communication disorders. (Now note that the theme of catastrophe and crisis has joined in.)

The major aspects of communication counseling were identified many years ago by Webster (1977), as follows:

- To receive information that the individual and his or her family wish to share with you
- To give information
- To help individuals clarify their ideas, attitudes, emotions, and beliefs
- To provide options for changing behaviors.

Note that this last point does *not* mean prescribing therapy or even necessarily advocating for a particular form of intervention. It merely means providing all of the information necessary for clients to make their own informed decisions from among the range of alternatives. (Here is the theme of recognizing the client as an expert.)

The intent of counseling with communicatively impaired persons and their families is to help them achieve the following:

- To grieve what has been lost
- To understand what has happened as fully as possible
- To develop coping strategies and to increase resilience
- To make peace with the disorder
- To make sensible adaptations to the disorder
- To capitalize on strengths in order to minimize weaknesses
- To live as fully as possible, despite impairment.

(All the themes are now mentioned.)

## What Is *Not* Counseling in Communication Disorders?

Although frequently taught together, counseling and interviewing have different goals and therefore are merely related processes. For example, a veritable chasm separates taking a case history from listening to a story and reacting appropriately to that story. *Interviewing* is the skill of finding out about another (in this case, someone with a communication disorder or a family member) through perceptive questioning and observation. In contrast to the counseling goals described earlier, the goal of interviewing is to provide the clinician with valid and pertinent information that informs the entire clinical process, including appropriate methods of intervention. This book is not about interviewing—it is about communication counseling.

Because the primary training of SLP-As is in communication sciences and disorders, not in clinical psychology or psychiatry, our clinical skills have implicit limitations and boundaries. Practically every specialized counseling textbook stresses the importance of placing some limits on counseling performed by the respective specialists. Counseling in our disciplines is no exception. The ASHA Scope of Practice statements for both audiology and speech-language pathology (ASHA, 2007, 2004) limit our counseling responsibilities to those that relate to communication disorders.

As counselors to clients with communication disorders, we are not clinical psychologists, and as is reiterated throughout this book, one of our primary sensitivities must be to know when our skills are not enough, and when referrals to other professionals such as psychiatrists, psychologists, genetic counselors, or social workers are appropriate. Box 1–1 lists some activities that can be considered outside the scope of practice for communication counselors.

In the remainder of this book, the term *communication counseling* replaces the rather burdensome phrase "counseling individuals and their families who have communication disorders." Use of this term should provide a continual reminder of the boundaries of our counseling work.

## Coaching

Coaching is a fast-growing new entry in the broad field of the helping professions and is relevant to communication counseling; thus, a brief note on coaching is in order here. Audrey has been trained as a life coach, but both of us practice many of its principles and tactics primarily in helping people (with and without language disorders) to age and to do it successfully, and in helping adult children to plan with and support their aging parents. The principles and skills of life coaching provide at least as pertinent a model for SLP-As as that on which more conventionally defined counseling is based. Coaching is a process that is grounded in wellness. Its emphasis is on normalcy and health, on correctly identifying sources of

---

> **Box 1–1. Outside the Scope of Practice of Speech-Language Pathologists and Audiologists: Selected Activities**
>
> As SLP-As, we do not have the background that would permit us to predict:
>
> ■ The outcome and course of recovery for Mr. A's aphasia
>   *We are not fortune-tellers.*
> ■ Whether Ms. G's next child also will have a hearing loss
>   *Not only are we not fortune-tellers, but also we are not genetic counselors.*
> ■ If Mark and Arlene's marriage will survive their child's traumatic brain injury
>   *We are not fortune-tellers, genetic counselors, or marriage counselors.*
> ■ What the course of Mrs. Z's Alzheimer disease will be
>   *We are not fortune-tellers, genetic counselors, marriage counselors, or neuropsychologists. Furthermore, no true professional would attempt to make such predictions.*

---

problems and teaching problem-solving skills to apply to them, and developing and implementing pertinent action plans. Coaching also focuses on differentiating those problems that are within a person's ability to control from those that are beyond such control.

## Process-Specific Definitions

### Who Practices Communication Counseling?

Who are the health-related professionals who practice communication counseling? The answer, of course, is SLP-As.

### With Whom Is Communication Counseling Practiced?

In identifying those persons with whom communication counseling is practiced, no term is entirely suitable. The word "patient" implies sickness. The phrase "individuals with speech, language, or hearing disorders" (much less "and their families") seems just too big a mouthful. So for simplicity, currency, and clarity, the term "client" is used throughout this book; thus, SLP-As practice communication counseling with their clients.[2]

## When Does an SLP-A Provide Counseling?

Communication counselors at times may set aside sessions for counseling their clients. An example of such sessions is the resilience and optimism-building workshop models described in Chapter 8. The counseling provided by SLP-As, however, is more likely to be accomplished "on the fly" or around the edges of more traditional therapy, during more communication-focused intervention sessions with adult clients, for example, when an aphasic man with inconsistent family support may express doubts about the value of this therapy for him, or when a dysarthric woman whose progress has failed to meet her expectations voices her disappointment.

These instances may reveal important relevant information, for example, that sleeping problems are interfering with concentration. Counseling also often gets tucked into brief parent or family encounters at the beginning of a session, before more structured treatment begins, or at its end, when we may be summarizing what happened during the session itself. A useful term for such mini-encounters is "counseling moments" (examples are provided throughout this book). As effective communication counselors, we must be alert for these moments and be prepared to practice our counseling skills in ongoing, small, and even casual interactions throughout more focused clinical interventions.

## A Note on Depression and Communication Disorders

It is necessary to be emphatic about the association between communication disorders and depression and learned helplessness (Seligman, 1975). Without exception, communication disorders

---

[2]In this context, it is striking how overwrought the language of this discipline is. This is rather ironic, because a basic belief of the profession concerns clear, concise, intelligible, and, for some people, even "functional" language.

potentially can result in reactive depression for both the affected person and family members. With disorders that involve brain damage, concomitant depression may be brought about by faulty or disturbed patterns of normal neural transmission. Finally, some clients may have come to their present disorder already depressed. Nevertheless, it is essential to recognize that counselors in communication disorders lack the technical skills and the credentials to treat depression, either behaviorally or pharmacologically. But because depression is so likely to co-occur with the catastrophic problems we deal with, it is extremely important for us to be highly sensitive to problems that forecast it. Although the newly released *Diagnostic and Statistical Manual of Mental Disorders, 5th edition* (DSM-V, American Psychiatric Association, 2013) has modified its classification of depressive disorders to some extent, the following still serve us well as characteristics of depression: mood disorders, lack of zest, unexplained weight loss, sleeping problems, psychomotor problems, excessive fatigue, feelings of worthlessness, and statements of futility. When these indicators are present, the ethical responsibility of the SLP-A is to state relevant concerns directly, make appropriate referrals, and provide adequate follow-up regarding implementation of recommendations.[3]

## Organization of the Rest of the Book

As noted earlier, Chapter 2 provides an introduction to positive psychology, which is the theoretical heart of this book's approach to communication counseling. Chapter 3 concerns clinical skills and specific techniques. The next four chapters focus specifically on counseling in communication disorders. They are developed according to a lifespan perspective. Thus, counseling in the context and perspective of parents of children at risk for or with communication problems in childhood is the first of these chapters (Chapter 4).

---

[3]Note that both authors accept mutual responsibility for all of the opinions in this book; however because we both often prefer to use personal pronouns, the "I" in the adult chapters is more likely to be ALH and the "I" in the child chapters is more likely to be RLN. But mostly we use Audrey or Ryan to disambiguate ourselves. The "I" that occurs in Chapter 9, refers to Stan Goldberg, who contributed that chapter.

Its focus is on working with parents and primary caregivers, in keeping with the principle that counseling without family "buy-in" will have only limited effectiveness. Counseling issues concerning children and adolescents with communication disorders are addressed in Chapter 5. Although many of the issues parents consider are similar, there are unique opportunities for productive counseling in our working with children as we assist them in meeting the aims of counseling described in Chapter 3.

Chapters 6 and 7 focus on adults. Chapter 6 concerns disorders whose natural progression is toward improvement (e.g., stroke, traumatic brain injury in adults, hearing disorders). Individual and group work is discussed for both individuals who have such disorders and their significant others. Chapter 7 concerns disorders whose natural progression is toward deterioration (e.g., Alzheimer disease, Parkinson disease). Chapter 8 presents some templates for workshops in resilience and optimism that can be adapted for use with families across the age span and for how to counsel individuals with communication disorders when time is the issue. Chapter 9, a gift from the pen of noted authority Stan Goldberg, provides insights into counseling for dying patients—an area that is virtually unmentioned in our field, yet one in which practitioners increasingly find themselves.

The "clinical" chapters (Chapters 4–7) are somewhat similarly ordered. Each chapter is organized to address issues that are unique in terms of the relevant information and counseling needs. We attend to both individual and group work. As noted previously, valuing stories and illness narratives is a critical part of the counseling process, so each chapter includes real stories about real problems providing everyday examples of a successful, positive, resilient outcome. Finally, each clinical chapter includes relevant learning exercises and formats for clinicians to use as practice. These exercises come mostly from our experiences in teaching communication counseling to graduate students.

There were significant, untouched topics in the first edition of this book. We wanted to more directly address issues associated with helping parents and families navigate the bureaucracy of systems and other areas of potential frustration. We also felt a need to more explicitly address communication counseling with children. Furthermore, the first edition did not cover issues such as counseling adult children of aging parents, attending to the specific needs of adults with hearing impairments, the issue of worries about mild cognitive impairment, or the specific problems of aging parents who have raised to adulthood their children with chronic disabilities and communication disorders. To the extent possible, we have tried to accommodate these issues here. Of note, the principles embodied in the "wellness" approach to counseling are relevant to all of these issues and can be straightforwardly applied in appropriate instances.

Counseling skills cannot be learned effectively by reading about them; rather, they are best learned through practice in constrained and nurturing environments, and through growing self-knowledge and introspection on the part of the learner. It is particularly critical for the SLP-A to think through personally experienced counseling moments and to evaluate them in ways suggested in this text.

The book's organization is based on the following assumptions. First, although a set of overarching principles is outlined for communication counseling, certain principles have more importance at some stages of the lifespan than at others. Such age specificity is a good reason for taking a lifespan approach. Furthermore, it seems unnecessary to differentiate a set of counseling principles aimed at specific problems. Principles that apply to counseling the parents of an at-risk infant (for example, helping them to become maximally resilient) apply across a wide range of disorders. Thus, each chapter presents a few disorders as illustrations or focal points, but the relevant techniques and skills have implications for the management of many other related disorders. These "focus disorders" are highly representative of the broader class of disorders that share their basic characteristics. Skilled clinicians rely on information concerning the facts of a given disorder, on community resources, and on the Internet. Such information itself is not inherent in the counseling process, but counseling certainly depends on it.

## The Formalities

Finally, it is necessary to discuss the formalities of counseling for our profession. The most important ones are differences between group and individual counseling, the timing of counseling, and its intensity; these are discussed briefly next.

## Group and Individual Counseling

A natural inclination is to relegate group counseling and individual counseling to two separate, mutually exclusive categories, each of which is restricted to use in specific circumstances or for specific clients. This view is difficult to justify, however. Both modes are effective, and they can even be undertaken simultaneously.

Our own clinical experience bears this out. Along with our commitment to shared expertise, we are inclined to favor group counseling. We like the notion of even more than two or three experts in a room. Short-term discussion groups and workshops for families concerning specific disorders provide an opportunity to promote and foster shared stories and problem solving. Skill-focused workshops on topics such as developing resilience or learning effective parenting techniques, or learning to change listening patterns and to tolerate hearing aids for older individuals, are excellent venues for sharing informational aspects of the counseling process.

Alternatively, there is undeniable value in one-on-one interactions as well, but much of this work, as mentioned earlier, occurs at the outset or conclusion of more direct intervention, or is nestled into such sessions.

## Timing and Intensity of Counseling

Whether it is with individuals or groups, counseling should begin in the earliest phases of treatment, when it is most needed. This is true across the age spectrum, from parents' initial recognition that their child is at risk, to the early days following a stroke or a diagnosis of Alzheimer disease or hearing loss. As mentioned earlier, providing information is just one of the functions of counseling, particularly early on. It also is important to remember that support and reassurance, as well as information, will continue to be needed as life with a problem is lived, but that the intensity of those needs should diminish; thus, counseling often occurs in those counseling moments described earlier. Finally, a point worth repeating is that counseling is more than just a set of skills to be practiced with clients; it also incorporates perceptiveness and an attitude of respect and sensitivity that permeates every aspect of every clinical interaction.

## Conclusion

This chapter provides an overview of a principled approach to communication counseling with a focus somewhat different from our profession's more traditional approaches. Although the SLP-A may view a leap into this relative unknown as a risky undertaking, the novel principles and techniques presented here are neither untested nor without application in other fields.

In the following poem, the rewards of maintaining an openness to change, despite its risks, are well illustrated:

"The Guest House"

This being human is a guest house.
Every morning a new arrival.

A joy, a depression, a meanness,
some momentary awareness comes
as an unexpected visitor.

Welcome and entertain them all!
Even if they're a crowd of sorrows,
Who violently sweep your house
empty of its furniture.

Still, treat each guest honorably.
He may be cleaning you out
for some new delight.

The dark moment, the shame, the malice,
Meet them at the door laughing,
and invite them in.

Be grateful for whoever comes,
Because each has been sent
as a guide from beyond.

—Jalal al-Din Rumi
*The Essential Rumi*, translations by
Coleman Barks with John Moyne,
1995. Reprinted with permission
from HarperCollins.

# References

American Psychiatric Association. (2013). *Diagnostic and statistical manual of mental disorders* (5th ed.). Washington, DC: Author.

American Speech-Language-Hearing Association. (2004). *Scope of practice in audiology.* Retrieved from http://www.asha.org

American Speech-Language-Hearing Association. (2007). *Scope of practice in speech-language pathology.* Retrieved from http://www.asha.org

Barnes, C., Mercer, G., & Shakespeare, T. (1999). *Exploring disability: A sociological introduction.* Cambridge, UK: Polity.

Ben-Shahar, T. (2010). *Being happy.* New York, NY: McGraw-Hill.

Chodron, P. (2001). *The places that scare you: A guide to fearlessness in difficult times.* Boston, MA: Shambhala.

Coles, R. (1989). *The call of stories: Teaching and the moral imagination.* Boston, MA: Houghton Mifflin.

Diener, E., & Biswas-Diener, R. (2008). *Happiness: Unlocking the mysteries of psychological wealth.* Malden, MA: Blackwell.

Frank, A. (1995). *The wounded storyteller: Body, illness and ethics.* Chicago, IL: University of Chicago Press.

Fredrickson, B. L. (2009). *Positivity.* New York, NY: Crown.

Goldberg, S. (2006). Shedding your fears: Bedside etiquette for dying patients. *Topics in Stroke Rehabilitation, 13,* 63–67.

Haidt, J. (2006). *The happiness hypothesis: Finding modern truth in ancient wisdom.* New York, NY: Basic Books.

Hinckley, J. (2006). Finding messages in bottles: Successful living with aphasia as revealed through personal narrative. *Topics in Stroke Rehabilitation, 13,* 25–36.

Holland, A., Cherney, L., & Halper, A. (2010). Tell me your story: Analysis of script topics selected by people with aphasia. *American Journal of Speech-Language Pathology, 19,* 198–203.

Kabat-Zinn, J. (2005). *Full catastrophe living. Using the wisdom of your body and mind to face stress, pain, and illness* (15th anniversary ed.). New York, NY: Delta.

Kazantsakis, N. (1996). *Zorba the Greek.* New York, NY: Scribner.

Kleinman, A. (1988). *The illness narratives: Suffering healing and the human condition.* New York, NY: Basic Books.

Kübler-Ross, E. (1969). *On death and dying.* New York, NY: Macmillan.

Lomas, J., Pickard, L., Bester, S., Elbard, H., Findlayson, A., & Zoghabib, C. (1989). The Communicative Effectiveness Index: Development and psychometric evaluation of functional communication measure for adult aphasia. *Journal of Speech and Hearing Disorders, 54,* 113–124.

Oliver, J. (1996). *Understanding disability: From theory to practice.* Basingstroke, UK: Macmillan.

Peterson, C. (2006). *A primer in positive psychology*. New York, NY: Oxford University Press.

Ram Dass. (2000). *Still here* (p. 185). New York, NY: Riverhead.

Reivich, K., & Shatté, A. (2002). *The resilience factor*. New York, NY: Broadway Books.

Robbins, T. (1980). *Still life with woodpecker*. New York, NY: Bantam.

Rogers, C. (1995). *Client-centered therapy: Its current practice, implications and theory*. Philadelphia, PA: Trans-Atlantic.

Rumi, J. D. (1995). The guest house. *The essential Rumi* (C. Barks & J. Moyne, Trans.). San Francisco, CA: Harper San Francisco.

Seligman, M. E. P. (1975). *Helplessness: On depression, development and death*. San Francisco, CA: W. H. Freeman.

Seligman, M. (2002). *Authentic happiness*. New York, NY: Free Press.

Seligman, M. E. P. (2011). *Flourish*. New York, NY: Free Press.

Shadden, B., B., Hagstrom, F., & Koski, P. (2008). *Neurogenic communication disorders: Life stories and the narrative self.* San Diego, CA: Plural.

Webster, E., & Newhoff, M. (1981). Intervention with families of communicatively impaired adults. In D. S. Beasley & G. A. Davis (Eds.), *Aging: Communication processes and disorders*. New York, NY: Grune & Stratton.

World Health Organization. (2001). *International classification of functioning, disability and health*. Geneva, Switzerland: Author.

# Chapter 2

# POSITIVE PSYCHOLOGY: IN BRIEF

## Introduction

Sam Schmidt was a race car driver who sustained a life-altering injury while practicing for the Indy 500 in January, 2000. As a result of the accident he became quadriplegic. But by May of that year, he had founded the Sam Schmidt Paralysis Foundation, devoted to research, funding and advocacy for people with spinal cord injuries. He commented in the *New York Times* (May 28, 2005) that the Foundation's work kept him from being depressed. He said, "I'd be thinking about what I can't do rather than what I can do." On the Foundation's website, Sam notes that in addition to medical research and to developing innovative rehabilitation equipment, he and the Foundation help others with spinal cord injuries to improve the quality of their lives. "I've come to understand why I'm here," Schmidt says. "We're spreading the message that you need to stay in shape and keep working hard, because something is going to come. Frankly, I've come to the realization that I'm helping a lot more people now that I ever could as a driver." He adds, "Let's face it, my motivation in the Foundation is somewhat selfish. It was started out of my desire to walk again, but if I can help myself and thousands of others achieve this goal, that would be fantastic!" It should be noted that Sam has other interests as well. He is co-owner of Schmidt-Peterson MotorSports, a well-respected racing corporation. Ritchie Hearn, who drove one of Schmidt's cars in the 2005 Indy 500, in the Times article commented that, "One of (Sam's) biggest things is showing people they have hope"

## What Is Positive Psychology?

To say that Martin E. P. Seligman and his colleagues at the end of the 20th century launched the positive psychology movement is an exaggeration. Many spiritual leaders (start with Confucius) and psychologists (include Abraham Maslow and Carl Rogers) set the stage. Yet it is relatively easy to trace its current ascendance to Seligman's presidential address to the American Psychological Association (Seligman, 1999) and its further explication by Seligman and Csikszentmihalyi (2000). Earlier, Seligman, with Stephen Maier and then Christopher Peterson, described the now-familiar concept of "learned helplessness" (Maier & Seligman, 1976; Peterson, Maier, & Seligman, 1993) and pioneered the concept of "learned optimism" (Seligman, 1998). In his 1999 address, Seligman charted a new territory for the scientific study of psychology. He noted that since the end of the Second World War, clinical psychology had shifted the bulk of its attention away from the task of making people's lives more fulfilling to the task of curing mental illness. Seligman contended that to be truly comprehensive, the discipline of psychology also had to concern itself with describing and enhancing mental wellness. Before we get to wellness, however, we begin this discussion of positive psychology with some comments about depression, the psychological disorder most commonly associated with communication problems.

Depression is more prevalent in the United States than it was some 50 years ago. Although estimates vary, the Centers for Disease Control estimated that 1 in 10 American adults have experienced depression (CDC, 2006, 2008). The age group with the highest likelihood of depression is 45 to 64 years (CDC, 2006, 2008). Lewinsohn, Hops, Roberts, and Seeley (1993) noted that approximately 20% of adolescents can be expected to have a major depressive episode during high school. This increase in prevalence among the young has occurred despite the development of more effective treatments, ranging from the pharmacologic to the behavioral. Thus, there exists the paradox of more effective treatment yet greater pervasiveness of depression. But why is that the case?

Seligman contends that psychology and its related professions have failed to emphasize issues concerning relative mental health, contentment, satisfaction, and the ability to enhance quality of life in favor of concentrating on ways to lessen mental illness. In the process, both scientists and the general public have become erroneously convinced that happiness is the opposite of depression. The truth is that the opposite of being depressed is just not being depressed. "Not depressed" is far from being happy, the stated goal of most individuals, including those who undergo formal psychotherapy for depression.

Seligman argued that psychology need not abandon its concern with mental illness, but that it should also focus a considerable amount of attention on the intensive and systematic study of what is right in human behavior. Scientific psychology also should include the study of how well-being can be increased. Furthermore, psychology should focus on how to help people build and increase their strengths and how to flourish, rather than concentrating specifically on how they can reduce and eradicate weaknesses. As a result of scholarly and research attention since 1999, positive psychology has enjoyed remarkable and growing influence worldwide. Chapter 1 has listed a number of these relevant works, and here are a few more: Aspinwall and Staudinger (2004); Fredrickson (2010); Lyubomirski (2009); Peterson (2006); Peterson and Seligman (2004); Seligman (2003); Seligman (2005); Snyder and Lopez (2005); and, above all, Seligman (2011).

Applications have been developed for both clinicians and lay audiences. Perhaps the most influential example is the earlier work, *Authentic Happiness* (Seligman, 2002), and the websites it has spawned, particularly http://www.authentichappiness.org and http//www.reflectivehappiness.com. Attesting to the growth of this movement, in 2005 the University of Pennsylvania initiated a master's degree training program in positive psychology; the Master of Applied Positive Psychology, or MAPP (see MAPP link on the University of Pennsylvania website), is geared to training psychologists, life coaches, and other allied health professionals in this aspect of the discipline of psychology. As another example of positive psychology's growing influence, when the first edition of this book appeared in 2007, there was only one course related to the issues raised by positive psychology among the departmental course offerings in psychology at the University of Arizona; currently, there are at least five.

When the first edition of the present book was written, the major thrust of positive psychology was on the emotional side of things, focusing on personal happiness. But as Seligman put it in a YouTube lecture (2011) positive psychology in recent years has grown from infancy, now taking a much broader focus on well-being. Seligman referred to the current stage as its "toddlerhood." Most recently positive psychology under Seligman's leadership has broadened positive psychology from personal life satisfaction to encompass the well-being and flourishing of society in general. This expansion should be welcome for communication counseling, since communication is such an unremitting interpersonal enterprise.

In this book we emphasize the personal and interpersonal rather than the societal aspects of well-being and flourishing; however, personal growth and change, and routes to achieving it, particularly in relation to disability, must be situated in the broader concept of well-being.[1] Being realistic about problems we face in our professions is a welcome and well-rounded change. The elements of this broader concept share three properties that Seligman believes "free people will choose for their own sake" (*Flourish,* 2011, p. 16) as follows: Each of these properties, he notes: (a) contributes to well-being, (b) can be pursued for its own sake, not merely to get any of the other elements, and (c) can be defined and measured independently from the other elements.

Selligman (2011) summarizes these properties in the acronym PERMA. The psychological, sociological, and indeed political implications are sweeping; PERMA can be seen not just as a goal for personal growth, but one that incorporates societal well-being.

---

[1]But be aware that this book is not only about ways to incorporate positive psychology ideas into our work with clients. It is also about ways to incorporate them into our own lives. Our credibility in this respect is that both of us (Audrey and Ryan) try to practice what we preach to clients, as well.

The acronym is explained briefly below and is expanded on later in this chapter. The elements of PERMA comprise the following:

1. *Positive emotion:* Ongoing positive affect, reminiscences and reminders of good things that have happened in one's past, and positive expectations of the future
2. *Engagement:* Absorption in ongoing activities, losing oneself in what one is doing, being truly "in the moment"
3. *Relationships:* Involvement with others, sharing, kindness, being there
4. *Meaning:* Belonging to or serving something bigger than oneself
5. *Accomplishment:* Pursuing and achieving a goal for its own sake.

It must be noted that positive psychology is not without its vehement detractors, most notably Erenreich (2009), who levels a number of trenchant criticisms at positive psychology. She sees positive psychology as implementing relatively shoddy experimental design and conflating relational and causal explanations regarding a number of issues in medicine, aging, and so forth. Seligman rebuts her comments in *Flourish* (2011), presenting a strong case for the importance of optimism and positive attitudes in relationships, in the management and outcomes of disorders such as cardiovascular illness (and presumably, therefore, stroke), and general issues in aging, but he agrees that the data on cancer (Erenreich's own disorder) are less clear.

## Positive Psychology and Disability

The recent realignment of positive psychology, moving from happiness to more general well-being, should be welcomed by clinicians who deal with individuals who have disabilities. Although the emphasis on happiness was a fine first step, in retrospect it needed to be tempered by concerns such as "Yes, but for some of us, whose life has changed, is happiness a meaningful goal?" There are many studies suggesting that dealing with negative experiences and unforeseen negative events can enrich and give meaning to our lives. Flourishing and well-being despite disability makes more sense than (smiley-faced) "happiness."

Seligman's addition of relationships and accomplishment (The R and A in PERMA ) is quite important for disability counseling, particularly for communication counseling. Relationships are very vulnerable to interference by communication disorders, as we all know.

The renaissance of interest in what is "right" about people already has brought about a number of relevant observations (described in detail later). Here, some reasons why positive psychology has particular resonance for counseling individuals with communication disabilities are reviewed. First, conditions such as difficult early-life experiences (Roberts, Brown, Johnson, & Reinke, 2002), physical disability (Elliott, Kurylo, & Rivera, 2002), and aging (Vaillant, 2002) do not necessarily have negative consequences, as is often assumed. Second, it is possible to describe and measure human strengths. Third, to a large degree it is possible to use personal strengths to increase overall life satisfaction and well-being. Most pertinent to communication counseling, people can be helped to develop resilience and optimism (Reivich & Shatté, 2002), as well as simple behaviors (Fredrickson, 2001; Fredrickson & Losada, 2005) that may enrich their lives. Skills such as these probably are crucial for everyday people to live successfully (that is, fully) in the wake of catastrophic events.

Positive psychology's emphasis on well-being fits nicely with our own profession's beginning attempts to break away from a disease model. It also appears to fit comfortably with a number of other recent issues and developments pertinent to communication counseling. These include the social model of disability, the expanded idea of who the experts are, the rising role of consumers in defining the delivery of health care, the growing respect for many forms of alternative medicine and approaches to counseling and coaching, and finally, the concept of change and how to accomplish it.

## Some Tenets of Positive Psychology

This section presents a brief overview of some basic tenets of positive psychology, with emphasis on those that seem particularly pertinent to counseling individuals with communication disorders.

For readers interested in further exploration, the extensive bibliography is useful. Many of these concepts are visited in more detail later in the book, as well. Because today's positive psychology has benefited by its concurrence with the "Age of the Internet," the bibliography contains references to a number of relevant websites, as well as books and articles. The following overview uses examples from clinical cases involving communication disorders to illustrate the importance of the themes of positive psychology. Tenets and beliefs are explored first, and then its elements in the order of the PERMA acronym are described briefly. Remember, as you read about them, that the current trend in positive psychology is to cast a broad societal net. Because we are concerned with interpersonal counseling in the niche of communication disorders, we focus on its more interpersonal aspects here.

## Positive Psychology Is as Concerned with Discovering Strength as It Is with Modulating Weakness

If communication counseling is to have a balanced focus on maximizing strength and modulating or compensating for weakness, then it is critical to look at both the disorders themselves, and at the strengths that individuals and families might bring to overcoming them. Clinicians must help their clients to discover, and then to capitalize on, their true strengths,[2] as well as to develop nascent ones. Here is an example of how this might work:

> Adama and Evan, who have just become parents of a child with Down syndrome, are surely devastated by this fact. Their catastrophe must be acknowledged. But what strengths do Adama and Evan possess that can be counted on to help them develop the resilience and optimism necessary to raise their baby successfully? Is Adama brave? Is Evan intellectually curious? Does either have a sense of humor and playfulness? How can these or other strengths be harnessed to help them manage the care and planning their Down syndrome child will need?

---

[2]Measurement of strengths and virtues is discussed later in the chapter.

## Positive Psychology Focuses Equally on Building on the Best Things in Life and Repairing the Worst

One goal of communication counseling that follows from the principle of equal emphasis on building and repair in life is that we play a part in helping parents, persons with disorders, and families to live as fully as possible despite their catastrophe. Here is a pertinent example:

> Joe and Sue had just begun their carefully planned and anticipated retirement life together when Sue had a major stroke that left her with moderately severe Broca's aphasia and right hemiplegia. It is crucial to hear from both of them how their best-laid retirement plans were left in ruins, and to honor the problems they face; however, the focus for the long haul (after suitable healing time) should be on what is still good. What pieces of their plans can be salvaged? What still works for them? For example, under these changed circumstances, how can they now take advantage of, and maximize, visits with their grandchildren? Can a travel agent experienced in working with disabled individuals be hired to help in future travel planning? Can an architect be found to modify the vacation home they designed years ago? How do Sue and Joe approach the architect and the travel agent?

## Positive Psychology Is Equally Concerned with Fulfilling the Lives of Normal People and with Healing Pathologic Conditions

A key assumption in the counseling approach presented in this book is that basically normal people are likely to be the recipients of communication counseling. This assumption has powerful repercussions for us as clinicians in the ways we approach clients. Thus, we do not have to be experts in pathologic denial, in transference, or in any of the traditions and variants of Freudian psychotherapy. We do have to recognize such problems when we see them, and to make appropriate referrals, but they will not dominate our interactions. The notion that we deal with generally normal people in catastrophic situations should normalize us, and help us to ask the right questions, listen appropriately, and provide wise, pertinent professional advice.

Some of our clients will have psychopathologic conditions, of course, and we have to be experts at recognizing such conditions and making appropriate referrals. People with longstanding bipolar disease, for example, are not immune to developing a communication disorder, or to giving birth to a child who also might develop one. Also, as previously noted, reactive depression, particularly for adults with neurogenic disorders, is quite common. But our own counseling job is much more strongly focused on normality in catastrophic situations than it is on psychopathology. The focus needs to be on "What's right with you?" rather than on "What's wrong with you?" and how our clients can use what is right about them to help them to manage their current catastrophes. Here is an example of how it might work:

Five-year-old Sean's parents are not particularly concerned that he is "slow in talking." Sean is an only child. His parents can understand most of what he says; he communicates "just fine" at home and has good social relationships in his kindergarten. The only reason they have come for this evaluation is that Sean's kindergarten teacher is very worried about what is going to happen to him in first grade. The evaluation reveals that Sean is a delightful little boy, very sociable and outgoing, but his speech is largely unintelligible. He shows remarkable ingenuity in communicating nonetheless. His hearing is normal.

He gestures, points, drags folks around, and is extremely responsive to prompts from others, suggesting minimal comprehension problems. Are these parents denying the potential severity of the situation? Will they benefit from counseling to help them develop insight into Sean's phonological problems? Such counseling probably is not a very effective use of their (or the counselor's or Sean's) time. Sean needs direct speech intervention, and his family needs to learn about language development and how they can harness Sean's strengths, as well as their own, to help with this process, that is, they need information and some understanding of the importance of their involvement in direct speech therapy. They need to be added to Sean's therapy team. Even from this brief summary, some of Sean's strengths, as well as those of his parents, are pretty easy to find. These strengths will be the counterweights to his problems and as such should facilitate therapy and the changes that Sean and his parents will be making as he enters a verbally communicating world.

## The PERMA Perspective

Having reviewed the basic principles of positive psychology, we now are in a position to explore the framework more fully. We do this in the order of Seligman's acronym.

### P: Positive Affect

One aspect of positive affect and its place in well-being and satisfaction depends on recollecting and savoring good things that have happened. For example, Joe and Sue (of the earlier example) report that in the past, they enjoyed cooking together, seeing foreign movies, and taking languorous vacations in the Caribbean. Could they develop a collection of their best recipes as a legacy for their children? Can they use subtitled films to work on Sue's reading? What could now be gained by putting together a long-planned scrapbook or a videotape of their previous vacations to Europe or Jamaica, possibly permitting them to savor their time spent relaxing there in earlier years? These notions probably can be built into direct therapy, of course, and not simply reserved for the communication counseling part of treatment. For our older clients, the importance of positive reminiscences is perhaps disproportionate to life's ongoing experiences, and to future expectations. In fact, it may be one of the most important parts of late-life satisfaction, particularly for our clients with disorders of downward progression (the topic of Chapter 7), where reminiscences have a major role for communication counselors working from a positive psychology perspective. They are discussed more extensively in that chapter.

### The Present

The second aspect concerns the pleasures of "present living." Included here are the satisfactions derived from activities as diverse as eating, talking with friends, and having satisfying sexual experiences. Little things, perhaps less obvious, also contribute to one's immediate sense of well-being (perhaps a pet's enthusiastic greeting at the end of the workday). The burdens of a handicapped child or the stress resulting from living with a partner with Alzheimer disease can, and do, intrude on present pleasures. Yet present pleasures have a terrific importance, and in many ways, they are under our control. Later in this chapter, there are some well-evaluated exercises that address this aspect of life satisfaction. All of them are appropriate or can be modified (see Chapter 8) for individuals/ families with communication disorders.

### *Positive Expectations for the Future*

The third aspect of positive affect concerns the future. The key here is to recognize and capitalize on one's own inherent resilience and optimism, or, through practice, to develop them possibly using some of the techniques referred to above. All of them are appropriate for our own practice, many can be practiced in their original form by our clients, and virtually all of them can be easily modified to accommodate many communication disorders. Parents and families of individuals who have communication disorders have immediate, lingering and often long-standing concerns about the future and what it portends for them, to be certain, but so do most people who are free of such problems. How shall we face the future? What current strengths can be mustered? What new skills can be learned to increase the ability to face what is ahead with flexibility, grace, bravery, and hope? How can we help our clients to learn them? One path is certainly by mustering and developing resilience and optimism.

Positive affect begins the PERMA acronym, but we have four other letters to go. It is not possible to equate a pleasant life and positive affect with "happiness" or with life satisfaction. In fact, some people who have few overtly positive emotions nevertheless are living fulfilled and happy lives, largely as a result of their engagement and their devotion to a meaningful life, their attachments to others, or their sense of achievement, however they measure it. Some well-known religious figures, such as the Dalai Lama or Mother Teresa, come to mind, but most of us also have some personal examples.

## E:  Engagement, Absorption, Immersion, Flow

All of us have, at some time, been so absorbed in what we were doing that time slipped away and we failed to realize that we missed making a previously arranged phone call or forgot to take the cake from the oven. Sometimes these experiences are annoying or frustrating. But there is also undeniable pleasure to be found in absorption. For most of us, the totally pleasurable experiences of losing oneself in a tennis or video game, or in a walk on the beach in the moonlight, greatly outnumber those episodes involving burned cake. Truly engaging experiences constitute the essence of "flow" as described by Csikszentmihalyi (1990, 1997). Engagement from the viewpoint of experienced meditators seems akin to being "in the moment" (Chodron, 2000; Kabat-Zinn, 1994). Haidt (2006) calls flow "the state of total immersion in a task that is challenging yet closely matched to one's abilities" (p. 95).

This temporary loss of a sense of time may be difficult to appreciate because often we are unaware of it when it occurs. But for artists and athletes, this sense of engagement and flow is unquestioned. For example, consider the samurai archer, who is at one with his bow—or, perhaps closer to home, Rafael Nadal on a really good day. Flow matters for more ordinary people as well, even though they may not be specifically aware of its value.

Unfortunately, flow and engagement may be among the first casualties for people who are beginning the process of dealing with the downside of their catastrophes. The mother of a child with disabilities who mourns the loss of time for herself may feel guilty about missing her time alone. She is unaware of how important engagement of this sort might be. Audrey recently heard a despairing description of such loss, as told by Mrs. J, the spouse of an aphasic man. Mrs. J perceived Mr. J as totally demanding of her energies as she helped him to carry out his prescribed after-stroke regimen: "I have to do everything, go everywhere with him. I'm not even alone when I'm sound asleep!" Mrs. J lamented the loss of personal control over the pace of her own life and, no doubt, the loss of flow. Jon Lyon (1998) notes about flow that:

> . . . all people need frequent and predictable periods in their lives when the actual act of participating in life dominates self-awareness, self-consciousness, even awareness of reward! . . . the

captivating nature of simply 'doing' the activity that causes its initiator to forget entirely about self, time, or outcome. (p. 222)

In communication counseling, we must pay serious attention to ways of reestablishing engagement, immersion, and flow in the lives of our clients and their families. For example, it is easier to find absorption in an activity that harnesses personal strengths. This is an important reason to identify such strengths.

## R: Relationships (Involvement with Others, Sharing, Kindness, Being There)

Relationships with others, from parents to peers to partners, are incredibly important components of communication, and therefore of communication disorders and counseling for them. Our disciplines have long recognized that communication is an intrinsic interpersonal activity, beginning with the fact that communication is not solely dependent on what one might intend by the words one uses, but how the meaning of the message is interpreted by the person who receives it.

There are, however, other levels of relationship, at least as important, that affect communication as well. Following the traditions of Erikson (1963) and others, Ryff, in her well-being scales[3] and her writings (see Ryff & Singer, 2001), and others, argue that positive relationships are essential to psychological well-being. Interpersonal problems are endemic to our fields. For children on the autism spectrum, difficulties with social relationships, from parents to peers, are emblematic. Social relationships can be negatively affected by almost every other communication disorder as well. This means that SLP-As must be constantly on the alert for the negative effects on social relationships and networks in communication disorders.

It is also important to point out that there are many bright spots as well. Resilience is a key here. Resilient people who incur communication disorders, either as parents or, in later life, as recipients of them, fare far better in the relationship department than those who do not encounter such problems. Of course, it is always

---

[3]Available on the Internet.

possible to learn resilience skills. Furthermore, in terms of aging in general, Vaillant (2002) points out that individuals who enter older age (when many communication disorders occur) with good social supports in place have the edge (along with some other features such as freedom from alcohol and nicotine abuse, and of course, resilience—termed gracefully, "the ability to make lemonade when life hands you a lemon.")

## M: Meaning (Belonging to or Serving Something Bigger Than Oneself)

Seligman's conception of a meaningful life is simply "using your strengths and virtues in the service of something larger than you are" (Seligman, 2002, p. 263). He further notes that this outside responsibility could be anything from family concerns, to allegiance to the Rotary Club, to the strict observance of religious practices. In the days following Hurricane Katrina, in the midst of reports concerning the devastation and horror in Louisiana, Mississippi, and Alabama, many instances of incredible bravery and outpouring of money, help, and services to the hurricane's victims also occurred. Here is an example, pieced together from a National Public Radio (NPR) broadcast at about the same time: The town of Lake Providence, Louisiana, a crushingly poor community of 5,000 in East Carroll Parish, opened its arms to refugees from Katrina's aftermath. One such refugee told a BBC reporter that after he revisited New Orleans to reclaim what was left of his life there, he planned to return to Lake Providence to live. When the reporter asked why, he responded, "Because good people live here." When one of those good local residents was asked how she explained the citizens' outpouring of care, fundraising, and support, she replied, "We are poor people here. We know what this feels like."

As more recent disasters mount, from Tohuku in Japan to Hurricane Sandy, so do examples of human and community resilience. Here is a blog from the New Jersey shore by Anne Mikolay, October 31, 2012:

> Resilience. It's everywhere. Whether it's senior citizens of Tomaso Plaza using old fashioned coffee pots to heat coffee on a barbecue grill immediately after the storm, or neighbors on Knapp Circle in New Monmouth sharing one generator, or Middletown Township arranging a special Halloween celebra-

tion for the children, or St. Benedict and St. Clement churches (and more, no doubt) collecting clothing for the needy, or Petco on Route 35 in Middletown opening despite lack of power in order to provide for four legged and feathered community members . . . New Jersey residents are rallying around one another. As New Jersey's native son, Bon Jovi, so aptly said, "We don't have electricity, but we have power." Kudos to Governor Christie for all he is doing. The big guy proved his mettle and then some. Regardless of your opinion of our Governor, he personifies resilience.

For families and children, as well as families and individuals whose communication disorders occur later in life, three themes are implicit in the foregoing examples: (1) What commitments to the meaningful life were in place before the catastrophe? (2) How can they be optimized? and (3) Can new commitments emerge as the result of this potentially transformative experience?

Following the Boston Marathon bombings, Audrey received the following e-mail:

> Charles Dankmeyer, a Vice President of the American Orthotics and Prosthetics Association, is spearheading a campaign to provide state-of-the-art prosthetics to victims of the bombings in Boston. Since some of the victims may be either underinsured or uninsured, the significant cost of top quality prosthetic limbs may be beyond the resources of these innocent victims. Thus, the AOPA has contacted both the producers of components for the prostheses and specialists who design and fit them for contributions to this effort. Dankmeyer reports that the response has been overwhelming and nationwide. Every patient will get the devices they need, and any cost not covered by insurance will be waived by the component producers and prosthetists. No one will be denied state-of-the-art prosthetics for financial reasons!

## A: Accomplishment (Pursuing and Achieving a Goal for Its Own Sake)

Accomplishment for individuals and families with disabilities does not seem to be the sort of thing that Seligman has in mind in his conceptualization of it, but he is completely correct in terms of its importance. Accomplishment is a double-edged sword: Parents' hopes and aspirations for their offspring may be dashed, or at least require reconsideration when their child is born with a problem that has long-term consequences. Similarly, hopes and plans for many wounded and returning soldiers can be seriously and permanently compromised by depression, head injury, posttraumatic stress syndrome (PTSD), or multiple amputations. Finally, many of the later-appearing disorders, such as aphasia or dementia, may require serious realignment of plans and dreams.

Look, however, at what "abled" individuals can learn from these individuals and how they deal with likely altered expectations and goals. One has only to observe events at Special Olympics or the Paralympics[4] to be overwhelmed by the joys of reaching one's goals by doing whatever it takes to succeed. There is no difference in the formula of the goal setting, motivation, and time and effort required to achieve goals. This is not limited to sports; it extends to excelling at a simple task once thoughtlessly performed but now requiring relearning or new adaptations.

What follows is an excerpt from Cynthia Kidder's beautifully illustrated book, *Common Threads: Celebrating Life with Down Syndrome* (Kidder & Slotko, 2001). The book is filled with stories of accomplishment by children and adolescents with that disorder, and it makes the point well:

> It was a tense moment in the Brighton Bulldogs locker room. . . . Everyone, sweating from the pre-game warm-up, knew that the winner had a chance for the conference title. They sat in uncomfortable silence. Suddenly, Derek Howes, a team manager with Down syndrome, walked to the middle of the room, clenched his fists and began to speak. "He started low," said Matt Stone, one of the varsity football players, "but then his voice rose in such a crescendo of "Go's, Fights and Bulldogs" that I thought his lungs would burst. His eyes squinted and his face turned red. He was more emotional than I have ever seen another human being in my entire life." It was the rally-cry, the pep-talk, the pre-victory cheer. Derek Howes had made

---

[4]Paralympics 2012 drew its largest-ever live television audience, except, unbelievably, in the United States, where events were only minimally covered. While few of us can ever hope to achieve Olympian standards, the efforts of these amazing athletes have potentially critical meaning and motivation for all of us, "abled" and "less abled."

his mission to fire up the entire pack of high-school athletes. "And when he was done," said Matt, "I was stunned. I wanted to laugh and cry and yell at the same time. The entire team erupted into a deafening cheer that only a football team can produce. Charging Derek, they gave him a giant group hug and then ran out onto the field. Needless to say, South Lyon never had a chance that night, and Derek Howes had earned a permanent speaking spot before every game. (Kidder & Slotko, p. 60)

These are the sorts of accomplishments that we must foster and attend to in our counseling efforts, not necessarily the big steps, but the self-satisfying smaller steps, for parents, children, and adult clients and their families. It is possible that upon his birth, Derek's parents felt bewildered, perhaps disappointed, and worried about their potentially denied dreams. But now imagine Derek's sense of himself, and his parents' sense of pride. It is no easy task to adjust or abandon lofty—and maybe unreachable, even without a disability—goals for one's children, one's life partners, or in many cases, oneself. But it is surely a task in which communication counselors have a role.

## PERMA Summary

The foregoing summary of Seligman's PERMA is seen through the specific needs of clinician-specialists in audiology and speech-language pathology. The summary is intended to lead readers to further reading, particularly the sources cited throughout this book. Readers are also encouraged to visit the various websites related to flourishing and well-being. A good place to start would be to visit, register, and then log onto http://www.authentichappiness. org and http://www.authentichappiness.sas.upenn.edu. These websites furnish a number of free tests that can be useful in developing self-knowledge to use in counseling. The tests can also be used by clients. Finally, they provide frequent updates on information on positive psychology that can be of personal and professional interest.

The ongoing development of positive psychology is truly a phenomenon of the 21st century, and countless websites, YouTube videos, and commentaries make it easy to stay current. The first edition of this book included a number of relevant websites, but since this is a constantly changing and updating process, this revision contains only a reminder to search the Internet frequently. But for starters, do look at the tests available to you for self-administration. Most of them permit readers to complete their own profiles and then compare themselves to a larger sample of individuals who share your demographics.

## Learning Your Strengths and Helping Others to Learn Theirs

Setting the boundaries on what psychological well-being might look like is an important step in exploring the basics of positive psychology. Also at issue, however, is developing a style of living in the world that capitalizes on using one's own strengths. Western culture encourages people to know their limitations, to seek self-improvement, and to live within their constraints. (Consider that as of 2012, Amazon.com listed 279,000 titles under the heading of personal growth, including three on writing self-help books.)

Far less attention has been given to recognizing personal strengths and virtues, and capitalizing on them, or using them to shore up some less-well-honed traits. A useful guide for finding personal strengths is the Values in Action (VIA) assessment available through the Authentic Happiness website mentioned earlier. This measure, developed by Peterson and Seligman, is the product of a principled attempt to provide a foundation in psychology for the scientific study of character and grew out of their book *Character Strengths and Virtues: A Classification and Handbook* (2004). Seligman refers to this book as an "un-DSM."[5] Peterson and Seligman, to some degree following the template that was used to develop the DSM, have produced a "Manual of the Sanities" (Peterson & Seligman, 2004, p. 3). The authors first explored a vast num-

---

[5]DSM , *Diagnostic and StatisticalManualof Mental Disorders* (referred to in Chapter 1), is a widely disseminated manual of definitions of disorders of mental health, and information on how to assess and, in some instances, treat them. The fifth edition (DSM-V) was published in spring, 2013. It is intended primarily for use by psychiatrists and clinical psychologists.

ber of resources, consulting a large pool of eminent authorities in human behavior and combing the world's philosophies, religions, literatures, films, and so on, for possible contributions to a list of character strengths. Next, they developed criteria for reducing this large data pool into a more manageable list of character strengths and virtues. At this step, they again sought input from their group of authorities. What finally emerged is a classification system designed to exemplify core properties of character, applicable across cultures and religions.[6] A list of these character strengths appears in Box 2–1. (Note that this list is really a "work in progress" amenable to change and modification over time.)

The list comprises seven core moral virtues recognized by the world's religions and thought to be universal. These moral virtues are temperance, transcendence, wisdom and knowledge, courage, humanity, and justice. Listed under each virtue are the specific traits that address the core moral virtues. Twenty-four traits are identified, each a trait for people to consider in relation to themselves as they take the VIA to find their strengths. No one will find that he or she is blessed with all 24 traits; in fact, the VIA concentrates on an individual's five most prominent ones, referred to as "signature strengths." Peterson and Seligman (2004, p. 18) note that such strengths (or personal traits) are the stuff of the "real me," "the strengths that one owns, celebrates, frequently exercises. And most of us know what some of them are."[7] A cornerstone of this book is that counselor-clinicians need to know themselves. (More on this precept is presented in the next chapter.) To apply positive psychology to communication counseling, it is necessary to become familiar with its exercises and approaches, an exploration that furnishes common ground for both counselors and their clients. Doing the exercises and taking the assessment test obviously also has direct personal benefit. Therefore, self-administration of the VIA (available on the aforementioned websites) to get a blueprint of personal signature strengths is a useful undertaking for all SLP-As. After completion of the VIA and review of the results, illustrating

---

[6]A highly recommended distillation of character strengths and virtues can be found in Peterson's *A Primer in Positive Psychology* (2006).

[7]"Signature Strengths Test" appears as the appendix to Flourish (Seligman, 2011). Audrey and Ryan recently took it, and it showed remarkable concordance with their most recent VIA scores of 2 years prior.

## Box 2–1. Character Strengths and Virtues

Strengths of Temperance
- Forgiveness/mercy
- Prudence
- Humility and modesty
- Self-regulation (self-control)

Strengths of Transcendence
- Appreciation of beauty and excellence (awe, wonder, elevation)
- Gratitude
- Hope (optimism, future-mindedness, future orientation)
- Humor and playfulness
- Spirituality (religiousness, faith, purpose)

Strengths of Wisdom and Knowledge
- Creativity (originality, ingenuity)
- Curiosity (interest, novelty seeking, openness to experience)
- Open-mindedness (judgment, critical thinking)
- Love of learning
- Perspective (wisdom)

Strengths of Courage
- Authenticity
- Bravery
- Persistence (perseverance, industriousness)
- Vitality (zest, enthusiasm, vigor, energy)

Strengths of Humanity
- Love
- Kindness (generosity, nurturance, care, compassion, altruistic love, "niceness")
- Social intelligence (emotional intelligence, personal intelligence)

Strengths of Justice
- Citizenship (social responsibility, loyalty, teamwork)
- Fairness
- Leadership

(Adapted from Peterson & Seligman, 2005.)

for clients how they might use their own strengths as fully as possible is easier. Relevant questions to ponder include the following: "How do I feel when I am using a top strength?" "How can I use my strengths in my professional life?" "How can I engage my strengths further, and what benefits might they confer to my clients?"

## Evidence

Many of the claims made by positive psychology have been addressed by relevant research. This section does not attempt to review all of the findings but rather presents appropriate examples to illustrate their breadth. Two areas are central to the practice of communication counseling:

1. The importance of optimism for developing and maintaining physical and psychological health and well-being.
2. The idea that happiness and optimism can be increased, which is central to the counseling model presented in this book. Although they are interrelated, they are discussed separately in this section.

### The Importance of Resilience and Optimism for Flourishing

As a prerequisite to considering its relevance in counseling, an explicit definition of resilience is necessary. Resilience is not just interior toughness, nor is it the ability to forge ahead no matter what, alone and against overwhelming, perhaps invincible, odds. Christopher Reeve remains a strong example of resilience, defined most rigorously in this way. But resilience also consists of factors that can be more prosaically embodied for most other people, who probably were never destined even to play a starring role in their high school play. Werner and Smith (1982) describe resilience simply as the quality that enables people to thrive despite adversity. This definition is expanded by Peterson (2006) and is operationalized in many activities adapted from Reivich and Shatté (2002), presented later in this book. Here, the focus is on a study reported by Charney (2005), who investigated American servicemen who survived imprisonment for 6 to 8 years during the Vietnam War. They found that servicemen who did not develop PTSD exhibited the characteristics that are presented in Box 2–2. A reasonable assumption is that the subjects of this research constitute a random sample of American servicemen, not supermen. But they were resilient, and resilience comprises these characteristics. In the words of Ann Masten (2001), such resilience probably is "ordinary magic." If it is a teachable skill, consider what it may offer to parents and families with communication disorders.

Many studies have examined the relationship between the qualities of optimism and resilience, and mental and physical health. In the context of physical health, research has shown, for example, that optimists live longer than pessimists (Maruta, Colligan, Malinchoc, & Offord, 2000), have healthier immune functions (Segerstrom, Taylor, Kemeny, & Fahey, 1998), and recover more quickly from bypass surgery (Fitzgerald, Tennen, Affleck, & Pransky 1993). Optimistic students visit their doctors less frequently and have fewer physical illnesses (Peterson & Bossio, 1991).

Regarding mental health, one of the most convincing studies concerns the role of resilience in older people who had experienced the death of a loved one (Bonnano, 2009). One of his surprising results was that almost half of the spouses he studied had

---

### Box 2–2. Qualities and Factors Associated with Resilience in POWs

- Optimism
- Altruism/helping others reduce stress
- Having an enduring set of beliefs or a moral compass
- Faith and spirituality
- Humor
- Having a role model
- Having social supports
- Being able to leave one's comfort zone (facing fear)
- Having a mission or meaning in life
- Having some training in mastering challenges

(Adapted from Charney, 2005.)

experienced no debilitating grief at all, and that an additional 20% recovered from their grief on their own. His resilient subjects did not lack feelings of sadness; rather, as Zolli and Healy (2012) point out, they demonstrated what these authors call "the capacity of a system, enterprise, or a person to maintain its core purpose and integrity in the face of dramatically changed circumstances." This certainly should pertain to many of our clients as well.

Similarly, optimists appear to be mentally healthier. A brief sampling of the relevant research supports this: Optimists are less likely to get depressed (Chang, 2000). Optimistic people have richer and more fulfilling social lives than pessimists (Diener & Seligman, 2002) Optimists age better than pessimists (Vaillant, 2002), that is, they have more satisfying relationships and are healthier and more contented than less optimistic people. Hollon and associates (2005) suggest that in cognitive therapy, one mediator of outcome is increases in optimism. Reivich, Gillham, Shatté, and Seligman (2006) found that in children, optimism also mediates the likelihood and degree of depression. According to Seligman (1998), optimistic insurance agents even sell more insurance. This is not to say that there are no negative consequences to a high level of optimism. Taylor and Brown (1988) have noted that mentally healthier people tend to overestimate the degree of their environmental control, see themselves in perhaps an overly positive light, and are sometimes unrealistically optimistic about the future.

Reivich and Shatté (2002) caution against such cockeyed optimism and instead suggest the concept of "realistic optimism" (i.e., maintaining a positive outlook without denying observable and verifiable facts, or ignoring negative aspects). Schneider (2001) discusses the "real world" issue of situations that permit latitude in how events are to be interpreted (she refers to them as having "fuzzy meaning"). She points out that denying or downplaying facts is neither helpful nor adaptive, and that optimism and pessimism both require caution and tempering. Aspinwall and Barnhart (2000) and Aspinwall, Richter, and Hoffman (2001) also suggest that optimists must not ignore negative information but rather use it as a barometer for changing strategies and as the basis for improving their performances. Nevertheless, the evidence supports the importance of optimism and resilience in flourishing and well-being.

The evidence also sets the stage for the applied work in building and fostering resilience in individuals. More broadly, it has put in motion programs that foster resilience and optimism in school children, strongly in place in both British and Australian schools, in addition to programs in North America. Most recently, Seligman and his colleagues have worked with success in teaching resilience skills to soldiers. Specifically, this involves educating soldiers about skills that contribute to posttraumatic *growth*, as opposed to posttraumatic *stress*. Strongly related to this work is the U.S. Army-sponsored program in effect since 2009, whereby the army's teachers, its drill sergeants, go through a rigorous 8-day training program designed to build resilience.

## Positive Emotions and Flourishing

The role of positive emotions (e.g., love, hope, trust, awe, enjoyment) and their importance in the good life were explored in the pioneering work of Barbara Fredrickson and her colleagues at the University of Michigan. Fredrickson's seminal contribution to the field has been to begin the process of explaining why the ability to experience positive emotions may be the basis of flourishing and thriving in a satisfying and meaningful life.

Specifically, Fredrickson and her colleagues have developed the broaden-and-build theory (Fredrickson, 2001, 2010). This theory posits that positive and negative emotions are distinctive and complementary.

Negative emotions (e.g., anger, fear, sadness) tend to narrow people's reactive abilities to those that have fostered survival. (Seligman refers to our "Pleistocene heritage" to describe them.) The "fight or flight" response is the primary example. Largely reactive (and not necessarily the subject of painstaking consideration, debate, and reconsideration), these behavioral automatisms have had an undeniable role in survival not only for our ancestors but also in many situations in the 21st century, such as Indonesia's and Japan's tsunamis, Hurricanes Katrina and Sandy, and the devastating earthquakes in Pakistan and Haiti.

Positive emotions, on the other hand, "broaden an individual's momentary thought-action repertoire and undo the narrow psychological and physiologic preparation for specific action" (Fredrickson, 1998). In the context of a wellness-based approach to counseling, broadened repertoires of actions include helping people to see the "big picture" and to help them to frame it in optimistic, positive nurturing terms.

Fredrickson's broaden-and-build theory posits that broadening provides a foundation for developing a person's strengths, including physical and intellectual strengths, as well as social and psychological ones. Fredrickson's hypothesis states that over time, positive emotions increase and become more extensive, consequential personal resources. Fredrickson's work with Losada (Fredrickson & Losada, 2005) looked at a large sample of subjects' reports of their experienced positive and negative emotions over 28 days. Using a nonlinear dynamic model, the investigators concluded that a certain ratio of positive to negative events was predictive of flourishing.

This ratio is very important. Specifically, Fredrickson and Losada found that flourishing (as well as positive emotion) results when positive experiences (even such simple things as receiving a compliment on one's work) and negative experiences (again, possibly as simple as hearing that one's work is sloppy) occur in about at least a 3:1 ratio, with the upper limit set at 12:1. This finding should give clinicians and counselors pause. We have been brought up on the notion that positive reinforcement is desirable, and Fredrickson and Losada's research to some degree substantiates this. But the negative consequences of overkill constitute just as important a finding. It is not hard to imagine that indiscriminate overflows such as "great," wonderful," or "cool" become meaningless to most people when clinicians deliver it at even a 10:1 ratio. As a result, broadening and building in the clinical context may fail to occur. ("Cheerleading" is neither broadening nor building.) These findings are particularly important for SLP-As if they aim to cultivate positive emotions in their clients to maximize health and well-being (Fredrickson, 2001).

## Exercises and Interventions: Evidence of Their Importance

Applied positive psychology incorporates many exercises and practices intended to illustrate particular points. These interventions also are learning experiences designed to teach new ways of thinking and new patterns of behavior. The aforementioned work on resilience training in the schools and the military is an extended example of such exercises. This book incorporates a number of the approaches that have been validated by research, as well as others (not necessarily from positive psychology) that are designed to enhance counseling skills. Box 2–3 describes five positive psychology interventions that were designed to increase individual happiness. These five interventions have been evaluated for their efficacy (Seligman, Steen, Park, & Peterson, 2005). Detailed instructions for carrying out these interventions can be found in *Authentic Happiness* (Seligman, 2002) and at the Reflective Happiness website. A few of them also are incorporated into later chapters of this book. Seligman and his colleagues made these exercises and a placebo control task available via the Internet and asked interested participants to practice the interventions according to the researchers' instructions. Randomly assigned to study and placebo conditions, individuals were tested before and after participation, and at 1 week after the posttest and then at 1, 3, and 6 months

---

**Box 2–3. Five Positive Psychology Interventions[a]**

Gratitude visit: Write and then deliver a letter of gratitude to a person who has been very kind to you, but whom you have never properly thanked.

Three good things in life: Write down three things that went well each day for a week. Include what you did to bring this good thing about.

You at your best: Write about an instance in your life that shows you at your best. Review the story daily and consider which of your strengths was/were involved.

Using signature strengths in a new way: After taking the VIA and receiving feedback concerning signature strengths, use one of them in a new and different way every day for a week.[b]

Identifying signature strengths: Note your five most pronounced strengths, and use them more often for a week.

---

[a]Studied in Seligman, Steen, Park, and Peterson (2005).
[b]A fine collection of ideas for implementing this intervention appears in Peterson's *A Primer in Positive Psychology* (2006, pp. 159–162).

after the posttest using the Steen Happiness Index (SHI) and the Center for Epidemiological Studies Depression Scale (CES-D).[8] The assessments were self-administered at the website. A total of 411 subjects participated in all of the follow-up assessments. The interventions "using signature strengths in a new way" and "three good things in life" resulted in increased SHI scores and decreased CES-D scores, with effects continuing for the entire follow-up period. The "gratitude visit" intervention produced changes that persisted for 1 month. The "you at your best" and "identifying signature strengths" interventions resulted in positive but transient effects on SHI and CES-D scores. The placebo treatment of writing about early memories every night for 1 week also demonstrated positive, but transient, effects in control subjects.

An important finding of this study was that although subjects were asked to follow the protocol for only 1 week, a substantial number continued to practice the exercises. Subsequent analysis of subjects who continued the exercises provided strong evidence that those who continued to practice the interventions showed longer term benefit.

Limitations of this research range from self-selection of participants to poorly defined participant characteristics. Nevertheless, it constitutes important work and provides justification for more widespread use of the interventions. SLP-As can use the exercises with family members without modification, although for communicatively disordered adults, relatively simple changes may be required. These interventions will be far more meaningful to the counselor if experienced personally, so all clinicians should perform the exercises themselves before asking their clients to do so.

Of note, precursors of these interventions, as well as a model for their use, have been influenced by work in cognitive behavioral therapy (CBT) for treatment of depression (Beck, 1973; Beck, Rush, Shaw, & Emery, 1979; Young, Weinberger, & Beck, 2001). CBT is an approach to intervention that is rooted in reality and committed to change. CBT traditionally uses various behavioral exercises and interventions geared to helping depressed persons learn to reframe their thinking into healthier ways, and to put this new thinking into

---

[8]Both instruments are available on the Authentic Happiness website, and the CES-D also is available on the CES-D website. Lower scores on CES-D are better, incidentally.

practice. A number of studies have supported the use of CBT in the treatment of depression and other psychiatric disorders, and a recent meta-analysis of its effectiveness supports such conclusions (Butler, Chapman, Forman, & Beck, 2006).

Evidence of the effectiveness of CBT in conjunction with the antidepressant fluorine in the treatment of adolescent depression is available (Treatment for Adolescents with Depression Study Team, 2007). Coming full circle now is evidence suggesting that some of the hallmark exercises from positive psychology have positive effects on preventing depression in some children and youths (Cardemil, Reivich, Beevers, Seligman, & James, 2007; Reivich et al., 2006). Finally, Seligman, Rashid, and Parks (2006) summarized two recent studies, on what they term "positive psychotherapy" (PPT), that looked at the effects of positive psychology interventions with persons who had unipolar depression. The first study showed significantly decreased depression; this improvement was maintained for longer than a year after intervention. The second study, which compared PPT with "therapy as usual" and with such usual treatment plus medication, resulted in higher remission rates in the PPT group. Seligman and colleagues concluded: "Together these studies suggest that treatments for depression may usefully be supplemented by exercises that explicitly increase positive emotion, engagement and meaning" (2006, p. 774).

Recognizing the value of interventions designed to maximize well-being (broadly defined) is crucially important to our work as counselors, but another responsibility for clinicians counseling from a wellness perspective lies in helping their clients to develop the skills that permit them to take a realistic view of their circumstances. Seligman and colleagues (2006) make a related point, noting that even though the emphasis is on using core strengths to solve problems, and using positive psychology's exercises and interventions to decrease depression, specific problems are never ignored.

## A Final Note

There are numerous videos on YouTube related to positive psychology when experts are asked a question distilled as "Okay Dr. Whoever, if you had to choose one simple way to increase well-being in people, what would it be?" The question is always answered similarly by everyone (most importantly, by Seligman himself) by implicating being able to express and accept gratitude. Because the first chapter of this book stressed the importance of narrative, Audrey shares a narrative here:

> My first VIA produced a ho-hum gratitude score. "Seligman noted in his writings that he learned how to be more optimistic." I thought, *Can I learn to be more thankful?* I, who seldom wrote thank you notes, expected none, seldom remembered to say "thank you" when I felt it was implicit on my part, went to work. Know what? It works!
>
> My last VIA score went up; it is now one of my strengths. But the truly amazing part is that I am a fuller person, for I learned in the process to accept gratitude as well. Recently a feral cat (I call her Pacha Mama) came to live in my backyard. I am interested in studying cat behavior, and since I will not hang around lions or tigers long enough to study them big time, I decided to observe this feral pussycat and learn about her.
>
> So I have been feeding Pacha, and hopefully, befriending her in my backyard. Food is certainly important, but she ate and ran. One recent morning, she was waiting with surprising enthusiasm. I took her food out to her and narrowly avoided stepping on a huge dead rat. Pacha Mama is expressing gratitude! A gift to me, unsolicited. I took it inside and deposited it in my garbage can. And then I cried. I have seldom felt such a surge of well-being and positivity.

## Conclusion

This chapter reviews the major tenets of positive psychology, particularly as they relate to communication counseling. The most important points are outlined, but more extensive and nuanced reading is necessary for complete understanding. A key concept is that there is great value in learning more about positive psychology, not only for clients but for clinicians and counselors as well. This is, after all, normal, not abnormal, psychology, and its benefits can certainly apply to counselors as well.

# References

Aspinwall, L. G., & Barnhart, S. M. (2000). What I do know won't hurt me: Optimism, attention to negative information, coping, and heath. In J. E. Gillham (Ed.), *The science of optimism and hope: Research essays in honor of Martin E. P. Seligman* (pp. 162–200). Philadelphia, PA: Templeton Foundation.

Aspinwall, L. G., Richter, L., & Hoffman, R. R. (2001). Understanding how optimism "works": An examination of optimists' adaptive moderation of belief and behavior. In E. C. Chang (Ed.), *Optimism and pessimism: Theory, research, and practice* (pp. 217–238). Washington, DC: American Psychological Association.

Aspinwall, L., & Staudinger, U. (Eds.). (2004). *A psychology of human strengths: Fundamental questions and future directions for a positive psychology.* Washington, DC: American Psychological Association.

Caldwell, D. (2005, May 28). Auto racing: Ex-driver becomes a driving force. *The New York Times.*

Beck, A. T. (1973). *The diagnosis and management of depression.* Philadelphia, PA: University of Pennsylvania Press.

Beck, A. T., Rush, A. J., Shaw, B. F., & Emery, G. (1979). *Cognitive therapy of depression.* New York, NY: Guilford.

Ben-Shahar, T. (2006, March 22). *Finding happiness in a Harvard classroom.* National Public Radio interview.

Bonanno, G. (2009). *The other side of sadness.* New York, NY: Basic Books.

Butler, A. C., Chapman, J. E., Forman, E. M., & Beck, A. T. (2006). The empirical status of cognitive-behavioral therapy: A review of meta-analyses. *Clinical Psychology Review, 26,* 17–31.

Cardemil, E. V., Reivich, K. A., Beevers, C. G., Seligman, M. E. P., & James, J. (2007). The prevention of depressive symptoms in low-income minority children: Two-year follow-up. *Behaviour Research and Therapy, 45,* 313–327.

Centers for Disease Control (CDC). *Current depression among adults: United States, 2006 and 2008.* Atlanta, GA: Author.

Chang, E. C. (Ed). (2000). *Optimism, and pessimism: Implications for theory, research and practice.* Washington, DC: American Psychological Association.

Charney, D. S. (2005). The psychobiology of resilience to extreme stress: Implications for the prevention and treatment of mood and anxiety disorders. Grand Rounds presentation at Mount Sinai Hospital. *Medscape Psychiatry and Mental Health, 10,* 2. Retrieved from http://www.medscape.com

Chodron, P. (2000). *When things fall apart: Heart advice for difficult times.* Boston, MA: Shambhala.

Csikszentmihalyi, M. (1990). *Flow: The psychology of optimal experience.* New York, NY: Harper & Row.

Csikszentmihalyi, M. (1997). *Finding flow. The psychology of engagement with everyday life.* New York, NY: Basic Books.

Diener, E., & Seligman, M. E. P. (2002). Very happy people. *Psychological Science, 13*(1), 81–8

Elliott, T., Kurylo, M., & Rivera, P. (2002). Positive growth following an acquired physical disability. In C. R. Snyder & S. J. Lopez (Eds.), *Handbook of positive psychology* (pp. 687–699). New York, NY: Oxford University Press.

Ehrenreich, B. (2009*). Bright-sided: How positive thinking is undermining America.* New York, NY: Picador.

Erikson, E. H. (1963). *Childhood and society* (2nd ed.). New York, NY: Norton.

Fitzgerald, T., Tennen, H., Affleck, G., & Pransky, G. (1993). The relative importance of dispositional optimism and control appraisals in quality of life after coronary artery bypass surgery. *Journal of Behavioral Medicine, 16*, 25–43.

Fredrickson, B. L. (1998). What good are positive emotions? *Review of General Psychology, 2*, 300–319.

Fredrickson, B. L. (2001). The role of positive emotions in positive psychology: The broaden-and-build theory of positive emotions. *American Psychologist, 56*, 218–226.

Fredrickson, B. L. (2010). *Positivity.* Oxford, UK: Oneworld.

Fredrickson, B. L., & Losada, M. (2005). Positive affect and the complex dynamics of human flourishing. *American Psychologist, 60*, 678–686.

Haidt, J. (2006). *The happiness hypothesis: Finding modern truth in ancient wisdom.* New York, NY: Basic Books.

Hollon, S. D., DeRubeis, R. J., Shelton, R. C., Amsterdam, J. D., Salomon, R. M., O'Reardon, J. P., . . . Gallop, R. ,(2005). Prevention of relapse following cognitive therapy vs medications in moderate to severe depression. *Archives of General Psychiatry, 62*, 417–422.

Kabat-Zinn, J. (1994). *Wherever you go, there you are.* New York, NY: Hyperion.

Kidder, C. S., & Slotko, B. (2001). *Common threads: Celebrating life with Down syndrome.* Rochester Hills, MI: Band of Angels Press.

Lewinsohn, P. M., Hops, H., Roberts, R., & Seeley, J. (1993). Adolescent psychopathology: I. Prevalence and incidence of depression and other DSM-III-R disorders in high school students. *Journal of Abnormal Psychology, 102*, 110–120.

Lyon, J. (1998). *Coping with aphasia*. San Diego, CA: Singular.

Maier, S. F., & Seligman, M. E. P. (1976). Learned helplessness: Theory and evidence. *Journal of Experimental Psychology: General, 105*(1), 3–46.

Maruta, T., Colligan, R. C., Malinchoc, M., & Offord, K. P. (2000). Optimists vs. pessimists: Survival rate among medical patients over a 30-year period. *Mayo Clinic Proceedings, 75*, 140–143.

Masten, A. (2001). Ordinary magic: Resilience processes in development. *American Psychologist, 55*, 227–238.

Peterson, C. (2006). *A primer in positive psychology*. New York, NY: Oxford University Press.

Peterson, C., & Bossio, L. M. (1991). *Health and optimism*. New York, NY: Free Press.

Peterson, C., Maier, S. F, & Seligman, M. E. P. (1993). *Learned helplessness: A theory for the age of personal control*. New York, NY: Oxford University Press.

Peterson, C., & Seligman, M .E. P. (2004). *Character strengths and virtues: A classification and handbook*. New York, NY: Oxford University Press.

Reivich, K. J., Gillham, J., Shatté, A., & Seligman, M. E. P. (2006, July). Penn Resiliency Project. *Executive Summary*, 1–20.

Reivich, K., & Shatté, A. (2002). *The resilience factor: 7 essential skills for overcoming life's inevitable obstacles*. New York, NY: Broadway Books.

Roberts, M. K., Brown, K. J., Johnson, R. J, & Reinke, J. (2002). Positive psychology for children: Development, prevention and promotion. In C. R. Snyder & S. J. Lopez (Eds.), *Handbook of positive psychology* (pp. 663–675). New York, NY: Oxford University Press.

Ryff, C., & Singer, B. (eds). (2001, March). *Emotions, social relationships, and health*. New York, NY: Oxford University Press.

Schneider, S. (2001, March). Realistic optimism. *American Psychologist, 56*, pp. 250–259.

Segerstrom, S. C., Taylor, S. E., Kemeny, M. E., & Fahey, J. L. (1998). Optimism is associated with mood, coping, and immune change in response to stress. *Journal of Personality and Social Psychology, 74*(6), 1646–1655.

Seligman, M. E. P. (1998). *Learned optimism*. (2nd ed.) New York, NY: Free Press.

Seligman, M. E. P. (1999). The president's address. *American Psychologist, 54*, 559–562.

Seligman, M. E. P. (2002). *Authentic happiness*. New York, NY: Free Press.

Seligman, M. E. P. (2003). Positive clinical psychology. In L. Aspinwall & U. Staudinger (Eds.), *A psychology of human strengths: Fundamental questions and future directions for a positive psychology*. Washington, DC: American Psychological Association.

Seligman, M. E. P. (2004). *Lecture notes*. Authentic happiness coaching course.

Seligman, M. E. P. (2005). Positive psychology, positive prevention, and positive therapy. In S. R. Snyder & S. J. Lopez (Eds.), *Handbook of positive psychology.* New York, NY: Oxford University Press.

Seligman, M. E. P. (2011). *Flourish: A visionary new understanding of happiness and well-being.* New York, NY: Free Press.

Seligman, M. E. P., & Csikszentmihalyi, M. (2000). Positive psychology: An introduction. *American Psychologist, 55,* 5–14.

Seligman, M. E. P., Rashid, T., & Parks, A. (2006). Positive psychotherapy. *American Psychologist, 61,* 772–788.

Seligman, M. E. P., Steen, T. A., Park, N., & Peterson, C. (2005). Positive psychology progress: Empirical validation of interventions. *American Psychologist, 60*(5), 410–421.

Snyder, C. R., & Lopez, S. J. (2005). *Handbook of positive psychology.* Oxford, UK: Oxford University Press.

The TADS Team. (2007). Treatment of adolescent depression study: Long-term effectiveness and safety outcomes. *Archives of General Psychiatry, 64*(10), 1132–1143.

Taylor, S. E., & Brown, J. D. (1988). Illusion and well-being: A social psychological perspective on mental health. *Psychological Bulletin, 103,* 193–210.

Werner, E., & Smith, R. (1982). *Vulnerable but invincible: A study of resilient children and youth.* New York, NY: McGraw-Hill.

Zolli, A., & Healy A. M. (2012). *Resilience: Why things bounce back.* New York, NY: Free Press

## Websites

http://www.authentichappiness.org

http://www.positivepsychology.org

http://www.reflectivehappiness.com

http://www.reflectivelearning.com

# Chapter 3

# GOOD COUNSELORS: KNOWLEDGE, SKILLS, CHARACTERISTICS, AND ATTITUDES

## Introduction

In Chapter 2, SLP-As are urged to explore their strengths and to consider how to apply them productively to communication counseling. Knowing how to deploy one's strengths is a foundation on which to build counseling skills. Nevertheless, there are other important principles on which successful communication counseling is built. The first principle is that practitioners of communication counseling must have an extensive knowledge base concerning the disorders with which they work. Together with the specific competencies that define a clinical knowledge base, "people skills" also are critical for successful clinical careers. Indeed, both speech pathologists and audiologists have written about the clinical relevance of "social intelligence" (whether or not it is among one's signature strengths) (Rao, 2006; Taylor, 2005). Technical counseling skills, such as active listening, affirming, and disclosing, also are crucial. This chapter briefly reviews the necessary knowledge base for communication disorders and related professional issues, identifies desirable "people skills," and describes the requisite technical counseling skills for SLP-As.

## Maintaining a Professional Knowledge Base

Competent management of speech, language, and hearing disorders depends to some significant degree on an understanding of anatomy and physiology. Counselors must understand what is normal or not and what specific abnormalities result in which particular disorders. Furthermore, many of the disorders and impairments we treat are caused by medical conditions that have more generalized effects and often overshadow the communication disorder itself. All clinicians must have technical, accurate, and current knowledge about the anatomy and physiology of any disorder that is the focus of their counseling. In addition, clinicians must have state-of-the-art knowledge of the clinical methods they employ, and must maintain best practices in relation to the disorders with which they work. In this context, "being knowledgeable" means integrating all such disorder-specific information into direct management of the communication problem.

In communication counseling, medical facts usually take center stage or at least they loom in the background like the proverbial 600-pound gorilla. Many of the counseling concerns faced by parents of babies who are at risk for communication problems, or of children who have already demonstrated problems, are part of a larger medical picture. That is, although communication disorders may look to be in the foreground to us, the background of the precipitating condition invariably is at least as big, if not a bigger issue, to the client. This also is true (almost without exception) of adults with late-onset disorders ranging from speech problems resulting from a laryngectomy for laryngeal cancer to language problems secondary to Alzheimer disease. So it is appropriate for clinicians to acquire and maintain a good general knowledge base of relevant medical issues to use in counseling clients with communication disorders. What follows is a strategy for obtaining the requisite information.

One way to start is with the less personal, more general medical factors that influence counseling. Although wide individual variation is to be expected, competent counselors work with people, not with statistics or group trends. They must thoroughly understand the medical background of each communication disorder. It also is important to know the limitations of medical knowledge concerning the disease processes at hand, and to be continually alert for potential medical breakthroughs that can influence communication counseling. What follows are a few of the major issues, along with examples.

## What Is the Time Course for a Given Disorder?

Communication disorders have varying time courses that, in turn, affect clinical management. Many disorders of both children and adults are chronic to some greater or lesser degree and remain so, regardless of the elegance of the clinical intervention. Helping individuals, families, and caretakers to avoid pessimism and to develop a more positive outlook is both complex and difficult for problems such as raising a child with a severe hearing loss or with cerebral palsy. Help for these problems must be moored to a realistic, long-term perspective. Communication counselors are often called upon to deal with questions concerning developmental milestones that reflect (or predict) normal development, or changes in speech or language that should occur simply as a function of maturation. Parents of at-risk babies face an uncertain future. In the case of adults, related questions concern the time frame during which spontaneous changes (both positive and negative) might be expected. Answers to these questions must be individually determined and can vary markedly.

Furthermore, available guidelines concerning the time frame for spontaneous change are only approximate and often controversial. A good example is the expected duration of spontaneous recovery following a stroke. Such issues challenge the counselor's skills. Nonetheless, having some secure knowledge available, as well as some understanding of the limitations of that knowledge, is a professional responsibility of the skilled communication counselor. For example, an unfortunate and largely inadvertent by-product of poststroke rehabilitation is that individuals and families often develop the notion that they are in a race against time. They assume that when time spent in intensive rehabilitation is completed, no subsequent positive change will occur. More subtly, families and individuals equate the end of progress with when benefits run out. Rehabilitation staff may sometimes unintentionally convey such messages, and current patterns for reimbursement of services certainly reinforce them. The idea that there will be no more gains, however, is depressing and, practically without exceptions, untrue. The communication counselor should address such time-related issues, which are revisited in Chapter 6.

Parents of children with a variety of potential developmental disabilities face parallel issues with the passage of time. When babbling fails to occur in the same time frame as that recalled for Claudia's older sister, or when the first words do not appear by 15 months, what does it mean? Is Claudia retarded? These questions worry even parents who believe their children are developing normally, but they are specially loaded for parents of children who have disabilities. Can catch-up happen? What if it doesn't? Can we meaningfully predict Claudia's future? Again, these are time-related issues that constitute fertile ground for counseling.

## What Is This Disorder's Pattern of Change?

Some neurogenic communication disorders, such as those associated with traumatic brain injury (TBI), improve over time; others, like those accompanying amyotrophic lateral sclerosis (ALS), have a pattern of progressive deterioration. Patterns of recovery or deterioration play an important role in clinical management and influence clinical decision making by the person with the disorder, family members, the referring physician, and the communication counselor. For the type of collaborative, shared decision making emphasized in this book, the projected pattern of recovery or deterioration often is a crucial piece of information.

Deteriorating patterns are seldom pertinent for speech, language, and hearing disorders in children, in whom the time course of development and maturation typically is positive, if sometimes slow and meandering. But exceptions do occur. For example, deterioration occurs in children whose normal development is interrupted by frequent hospitalizations for ongoing medical problems, or in apparently normally developing 2-year-olds with a late-developing autism spectrum disorder (Rogers, 2004). In such cases, the counseling issues may have much longer trajectories, but parental concerns resemble those of a family in which an adult member incurs a disorder such as Alzheimer disease.

## What Problems Accompany and Influence the Disorder?

Many speech, language, and hearing disorders are accompanied by other problems that can influence counseling, as well as direct language and speech intervention. For example, in the case of right hemisphere stroke, the effect of anosognosia and neglect on language and speech can be substantial. Depression also is common in communication disorders, and parents and partners of the affected person are at risk as well. As noted earlier, communication counselors must be particularly alert to this possibility.

Pharmacologic interventions often have a profound effect on communication and such effects need to be well understood and anticipated. Communication counselors must pay particular attention to the effects of antiepileptic medications on children who are prone to seizure disorders. Some antiepileptic drugs (AEDs) also may have primary effects on communication. For example, topiramate is reputed to have negative effects on language, particularly affecting word-finding skills, in children (Kockelmann, Elger, & Helmstaedter, 2004). Adults with brain damage are especially vulnerable to antipsychotic medications, which are likely to affect cognition negatively (Maguire, 2000). For further information concerning pharmacology and communication, recommended reading includes works by Vogel, Carter, and Carter (1999), Johnson and Jacobson (1998), and Golper (1992). The communication counselor must be alert to the range of medication-associated problems. Particularly in these times of rapidly changing knowledge concerning the human genome, new pharmacological treatments emerge each year, and it is imperative for communication counselors to stay current. In addition, it must be noted that few texts in this area of communication disorders are particularly current. An exception is Campbell's handbook on ototoxicity for audiologists (2006).

Finally, many communication disorders are accompanied by motor, cognitive, and emotional factors and, furthermore, they often occur in complex social situations. Consider, for example, the myriad problems faced by children with cerebral palsy, TBI, or autism. Communication counselors must be able to place the speech, language, or hearing disorder in proper perspective when it comes embedded in a tangled package of problems, some directly affecting children, others directly affecting parents and thereby indirectly affecting children.

## Are Expectations Appropriate?

Communication counseling is enhanced when family, client, and clinician all have well-grounded expectations. Effective counseling depends on the clinician's awareness of probable outcomes for a given disorder. Parents, families, or individual clients need to have realistic and modulated, but nonetheless positive, expectations. For example, knowing that glioblastoma multiforme is a particularly virulent tumor tempers both how to counsel individuals and their families about the communication problem it brings and how to approach rehabilitation. The following scenario illustrates some of the considerations that may arise:

> Lily was a beautiful, buoyant 14-year-old girl who developed a fast-growing glioblastoma. Worried about her worsening anomia, Lily and her parents decided to follow her neurosurgeon's advice to consider language therapy. Both parents believed that the quality of Lily's life, however short, could be enhanced by positive, forward-looking interactive activities with a sensitive clinician. Accordingly, once-weekly therapy was undertaken for the 3 months that preceded her death. Counseling was an integral part of Lily's speech therapy.
>
> Even as Lily lost ground, she continued to smile, to worry about her appearance, and to anticipate the weekly visits and the carefully orchestrated conversations with her clinician. Her parents made the decision for intervention with a full understanding of the facts of Lily's disorder. It was part of their commitment to help her live her remaining days with hope. Another family facing the same problem, but with a different agenda and in different circumstances, could easily have made a different decision, with equal justification.

# Related Professional Competence Issues

Two additional areas of importance in a discussion of professional competence are: (1) the referral process and (2) knowledge about community and Internet resources.

## Referral Issues

As noted in Chapter 1, clinicians sometimes have difficulty with the boundaries between communication counseling and counseling for accompanying problems. Some clinicians face this boundary issue with queasiness; others scurry away altogether. For ethical reasons, communication counselors must recognize when the client's problem is beyond the scope of SLP-A clinical practice. The irony is that for communication counselors, this challenge is complicated by the very nature of their skills, particularly with adult clients who have language disorders. The "talking therapies" all revolve around just that—talking. Even when the problems are beyond their expertise, communication counselors are likely to understand the language and speech used to express them. Conversely, counselors and therapists from other professions face a significant barrier when attempting to help disordered individuals who have substantial communication disorders.

Skillful counselors respect the boundaries and limitations of their counseling skills and responsibilities. They also must know how to seek information from fellow professionals (particularly psychologists or social workers) and determine if co-treatment is an option. Finally, they must have a comprehensive understanding of a given community's referral resources for persons with communication disorders and know how to use the referral process. Developing such a database takes extensive exploration and networking with relevant professionals in one's community, but, in the long run, it pays off in more efficient and appropriate referrals.

## Information About Community and Internet Resources

In additional to professional referral sources, competent counselors also know about general community resources, such as senior citizen centers, access to public transportation for people with disabilities, disorder-specific support groups, experimental clinical and research programs, and so forth. Internet resources are of growing importance, and websites are available for all of the disorders discussed in this book. Comprehensive summaries of these rich and varied sources of information are available; the website Net Connections for Communication Sciences and Disorders (given at end of chapter) is an excellent and frequently updated source.

Programs that facilitate access to the Internet for people with neurogenic communication disorders and their families are becoming increasingly available (Worrall & Egan, 2000). The competent counselor knows about these resources and also about many excellent self-help books and personal accounts that can enhance counseling efforts. One of the strengths of Internet resources, of course, is that they are in a state of almost constant flux, with almost constant updating. This is exciting, to be sure, but keeping up is crucial and often frustrating.

## Personal Metaphors, Characteristics, and Attitudes

We begin our exploration of characteristics and attitudes with a brief discussion of the power of a personal metaphor for one's clinical life. Holland (2012), following the model of Ylvisaker and Feeney (1998), described the value of developing a personal metaphor as a unifying construct for characterizing competence as a clinician. Ylvisaker and Feeney argued that the process of developing self-understanding and applying it to clinical practice benefits from having a metaphor of ourselves as clinicians and then using that metaphor as a way to organize and judge our own clinical work. Developing a metaphor that resonates with oneself is not easy; typically it takes a bit of soul-searching. Clinical metaphors can stand anywhere along a continuum of helping—from coach to advocate to fairy godmother, to animal trainer, teacher, and so forth When a metaphor satisfies you, it should fit with how you go about the job of being a competent clinician. It will reflect your own values and beliefs; however, at some point a metaphor might not resonate with you anymore, and you might want to find a new one. For example, if you initially see the techniques of changing speech, hearing, and language behavior as being in line with how we might train Fido to roll over (i.e., clinician as an animal trainer), then that might seem like a good metaphor.

It is likely that experience will change your view, and perhaps Miracle Max of "Princess Bride" fame, who changes everything with a swoosh of a wand, may fit you better. So you change the metaphor; however, metaphors like both of those are probably too simple, and others, such as guardian angel, or coach, may be more descriptive of your clinical life. But it is always worthwhile to develop a metaphor and use it as your guide, and as a standard for judging your own life as a clinician. Keep the metaphor concept in mind as we explore characteristics and attitudes next. (By the way, neither of us will share our clinical metaphors with our readers, but it might be fun for you to speculate about them!)

## Competent Counselors: Personal Characteristics

In his text on clinical skills in speech-language pathology, Goldberg (1997) notes that lists of characteristics suffer from their lack of operational definitions. Nonetheless, some of these word pictures set the tone of what it means to be an effective clinician. Rogers' (1965) notion of unconditional positive regard for one's clients has always been a foundation, if not a mantra, for our own clinical practice, however lacking in operationalism it may be. Satir's (1967) compilation of desirable characteristics for clinicians who provide conjoint family therapy has a special resonance for communication counseling. The most relevant characteristics are listed in Box 3–1.

The issue of personal characteristics of effective communication counselors can be approached in a number of ways. Because self-knowledge is such a fundamental characteristic of good counselors, looking at one's own strengths is a good place to begin, as has already been suggested. This section presents some basic questions about personal qualities that appear to be central to effective counseling. The questions and elaborations provided are neither overwhelming nor comprehensive; they simply illustrate some personal characteristics that help people to be good counselors. Evaluate yourself in relation to them, and study the rationales for each characteristic.

---

**Box 3–1. Some Characteristics of Successful Clinicians**

- Reveal yourself clearly to others.
- Be in touch with your feelings and capabilities.
- Regard each person as unique.
- Differences are learning experiences, not threats or signals for conflict.
- Understand clients for who they are, not how you wish them to be.
- Understand that clients are responsible for their own behaviors.

---

(Adapted from Satir, 1967.)

---

## Are You a Good Listener?

Most counseling texts stress the importance of being a good listener. But what are the qualities of a "good listener"? Good listeners listen actively and nonjudgmentally. The futurist Elisabet Sahtouris has remarked that good listening involves "willingness to have one's mind changed by what one hears" (E. Sahtouris, personal communication, 2006). We certainly concur.

Good listeners are alert not only to what is being said but to what underlies the comments, what motivates them, and what meanings they have for the speaker. Theodore Reik (1948) referred to this process of listening both to surface and latent content of a message as "listening with the third ear." It is true that some people are born listeners, but listening skills also are teachable and learnable. Finally, good listeners know that listening is active. For one thing, "meaning" is not inherent in the speaker's words, but it is an active, co-constructive process, with the listener a crucial interpretive role. (See Goodwin, 2003, for a particularly well-reasoned example from aphasic conversation.) So when you hear someone saying, "I didn't do anything, I just listened," you should now recognize the inherent contradiction: The concept of "just listening" cannot coexist with the active process required. Some listening exercises are presented in Box 3–2.

## Box 3–2. Two Exercises in Listening

### Exercise 1: Listening for Surface and Latent Content

A. Listening requires active attending to what is being said and then responding appropriately. Listening involves being aware that content can be transmitted at two levels, that is, the manifest and the latent; one must listen for both. Finally, listening also involves being aware of both nonverbal and verbal behavior and searching for mismatches and congruities between them. Putting yourself on the sending end of this process, list six ways in which a person might communicate the following message: "I don't want to talk about this anymore."

B. For each of the following messages, identify one or more possible beneath-the-surface meanings:

- Ellen comments, "Oh, you like horror movies . . . that's interesting," while simultaneously swiveling her body away from, and breaking eye contact with, Rob, her conversational partner.
- George comments, "It's really hard to listen to Grandma because she talks constantly."
- Nora says, "You look great in that dress. I wish I also could wear clothes designed for younger women."

### Exercise 2: Latent Message and Locus of Responsibility

In each of the following requests for repair, what is the latent message? Where is the locus of responsibility? Why does it matter?

- "I wish you would speak a bit louder."
- "I'm afraid this is not one of my good listening days. I missed that."
- "Could you go over that again?"
- "Let's see if I got that."
- "It would be much easier for me if you spoke slowly and clearly."

## Are You an Active, Constructive Responder?

Gable, Reis, Impett, and Asher (2004) provide an excellent model for maximally effective responding to what one has been listening. Although their work centered on relationships among partners and responses to positive events, their findings have strong implications for parenting, counseling, and negative events as well.

The following positive hypothetical example concerns an 11-year-old client with diagnosed speech-language impairment (SLI):

> Mackenzie tells you that her poster concerning safety issues for children won the school's top award.

According to Gable and associates (2004), responses to such events can take one of four possible forms:

- Active constructive responding: "That's great! I bet you'll be doing more good art after this."
- Active destructive responding: "Don't get too carried away. Now they'll expect you to enter all the contests."
- Passive constructive responding: "That's swell."
- Passive destructive responding (a response that signals your lack of interest in or regard for the person): "I didn't know you could draw."

Gable and colleagues' (2004) data on response patterns of married couples indicate that active constructive responses predominate in good marriages. When any of the other response types predominates, less satisfying marriages are the result. The use of active constructive responding has much bigger implications, however. There is no doubt that active constructive responding is not always appropriate (for example, if Mackenzie tells you that you are a jerk). Gable and associates (2004) suggest that for strong effects, active constructive responses need to occur along with other responses, such as passive constructive, passive negative, and active negative responses in a ratio greater than 3:1.

How do the four response types stack up for negative events?

> Mackenzie reports her bitter disappointment over not winning the contest:

■ Active constructive responding: "I am so sorry to hear that. It must feel really awful, especially because you are such a good artist. But we have to figure out how to do better next time."

■ Active destructive responding: "I guess Jill is just a better artist than you are."

■ Passive constructive responding: "You are feeling pretty bad."

■ Passive destructive responding: "It was just a school contest, after all."

Many of us have been inculcated with the notion that neutral, reflective, nondirective responding is preferred in clinical interaction. In the foregoing scheme, this type of responding is passive constructive. Although this kind of response may be meaningful in psychotherapeutic interactions, the active constructive approach seems a better fit with the counseling roles and responsibilities of SLP-As. Box 3–3 provides some opportunities to explore all four types of responding, for both positive and negative reports.

## Are You a Good Communicator?

It is not necessary, and probably not desirable, for counselor-clinicians to aspire to be eloquent; rather, being a good communicator in this context refers to the ability to reach clients or family members on their terms and at their level of understanding, and to communicate with body language as diverse as getting down on the floor with a small child or holding the hand of a grieving spouse. Box 3–4 provides some practice exercises for translating professional jargon to families and patients.

## Can You Listen Comfortably to People Who Have Trouble Talking?

The very nature of communication disorders makes listening even more basic for SLP-As than it is for counselors in other disciplines, primarily because reduced intelligibility often presents an additional challenge. How do you handle situations in which you might

### Box 3–3. Exercise: Clinical Response Types

For each of the following clinical scenarios, provide an active-constructive, an active-destructive, a passive-constructive, and a passive-destructive response to both the positive and negative comments.

The client is Sybil, a young woman with mild TBI. She reports:

"I think I got the part-time job I applied for."

"I don't think I got that part-time job."

The client is Ned, the father of 8-year-old Teddy, who stutters. He comments:

"Teddy got picked to start the Little League game on Saturday."

"Teddy wasn't selected to start the Little League game on Saturday.

The client is Elise, spouse of Wilton, who has chronic dysphagia. She says:

"We had two couples over for dinner, and it was a disaster."

"We had two couples over for dinner, and it went just fine."

The client is Geoff, who has severe presbycusis. He says:

"The new hearing aids work just fine. I heard the sermon at church, for a change."

"The new hearing aids are as bad as the old ones. I still can't hear the sermon."

fail to understand what is being said to you, regardless of how actively and patiently you are listening? How easy is it for you to admit that you do not understand? How comfortable can you make the speaker whose speech intelligibility is an issue?

Because intelligibility can be a challenging problem, one interesting way to practice listening skills is by eavesdropping on fellow

---

**Box 3–4. Exercise: Translating Professional Jargon**

Put the following statements into common English:

"In addition to his difficulty with auditory comprehension, Mr. J seems to me to have a severe limb apraxia."

"Johnny's sensorimotor skills seem to lag behind his cognitive abilities."

"We are going to have to be very careful about the consistency of Mrs. S's oral intake, in order to avoid having her aspirate."

"I really think that the low intensity of Mr. T's speech contributes disproportionately to his lack of intelligibility."

"It is not uncommon for children who have phonological processing disorders become dyslexic as they mature."

---

clinicians and their clients and second-guessing their communication problems and solutions. Another solution is to develop a repertoire of graceful ways to admit lack of understanding in advance and use them when needed. "Faking it" is truly not an option. Almost all of us have tried it at one point or another; however, once caught by your client, you probably will not want to try it again. It is costly in terms of rapport, and your own embarrassment takes a toll, too. Here is an example:

**Client:** (*Unintelligible sentence*)

**Clinician:** (*Hoping to move on*) "Sure, that sounds like a good idea."

**Client:** (*Dysarthrically*) "What I say?" (Incidentally, the client's latent message is "Gotcha!")

Similar client interactions, with resulting professional embarrassment, have no doubt ensnared every clinician at least once. Box 3–5 provides some practice on how to handle such situations.

> **Box 3–5. Exercise: Talking to Clients**
> **Who Are Difficult to Understand**
>
> You are talking with your client, Bunny, a person of the opposite sex (from you) who has moderate executive system dysfunction and severe dysarthria following a TBI. Bunny asks you a question that you do not understand, but you say "yes" anyway. Bunny then says (intelligibly): "What did I ask you?" What do you say?

## Can You Listen to Emotions?

Communication problems inevitably have emotional consequences, often including crying and sadness, frequently realized in tears. In addition, some disorders (e.g., strokes) may bring inadvertent crying or laughing as a result of brainstem involvement. The one inviolate rule is that crying should be acknowledged.

Clinical viewpoints vary on the form of such acknowledgment. As borne out in our own clinical experience, helpful and authentic responses may include gently taking a hand, offering a tissue, and encouraging verbal expression of the emotion behind the tears. Such behavior is in fact part of the listening process, and crying is to be honored as something the client is willing to share. Regardless of how the individual SLP-A decides to deal with crying, all counselors should have a few alternative responses to use in clinical practice. The following scenario illustrates possible adverse consequences of lack of such a plan:

> A student clinician was summarizing the results of a long afternoon of exhaustive testing for a client with aphasia, who probably was confronting the magnitude of his language problem for the first time, and who also was fatigued from his efforts in the testing process. His wife was present. As the clinician was listing his problems and telling him about the long therapy road ahead, he burst into tears. The student clinician continued her report matter-of-factly, ignoring both the man's tears and his wife's concern. At the end of her litany

she asked, "Are there any questions?" When no questions were forthcoming, she stood, they stood, and all left the room.

Her clinical supervisor greeted them in the hall and attempted to ameliorate the situation. Later, when the supervisor asked the student why she had ignored the emotional scene, the student replied, "I didn't know what to do. In the American culture, men are not supposed to cry, and I decided that the best way to help him was to pretend I didn't notice!"

Besides tears, clinicians also have to listen to overtly negative emotions. Communication counseling can involve anger, frustration, and anxiety. Some of us can handle these emotions with equanimity; for others, they are very threatening. Of note, the anger, frustration, and anxiety are almost without exception never about *you*. It is more likely that they find their way to you because something else altogether has triggered a client's negativity and you were near. Alternatively (and ironically), you may have engendered enough trust to permit the client to feel safe about sharing negative things with you. When the negative emotions fly, take a deep breath while trying to remember that they are not about you. Box 3–6 presents some exercises for you to use to explore these issues on your own.

## Can You Listen to Ideas That Conflict with Your Values?

In clinical practice, communication counselors are likely to encounter people whose values and attitudes differ markedly from their own. Value differences can arise in relation to almost any controversial issue, from religious practices to sexual orientation. Attempting to change people's values, even when they are personally repugnant to you, is absolutely beyond the scope of clinical practice.

Values also affect issues that seem less controversial, such as the importance of speech therapy or hearing aids. Our professional culture views them as necessary in many cases, and probably even imperative. Clients may see things differently. How do value differences affect our ability to make and maintain clinically useful contact? Satir's earlier-quoted notion of accepting "who they are" rather than "how we might wish them to be" has important implications for communication counseling.

---

**Box 3–6. Exercise: Fielding Negative Emotions**

For each of the following client comments projecting discomfort or distress, provide a helpful and appropriate response:

"It makes me wonder about the genes on my wife Linda's side of the fence. I know for certain that nothing like this has ever happened in *my* family before."

"If you're gonna be my therapist, you'd better get to know me a bit. I smoke, and I don't want to hear about it. I also don't want you to be on my case for swearing. You can just forget that little goody-two-shoes routine if you work with me, honey."

"You're just like all the rest! Nobody around here tells me anything that is helpful! I am sooooo frustrated about what's happening! I don't even know what the plans are for next week! Does every parent with a TBI kid get such treatment, or am I special?"

"Is this for real, or what? The doctor says he's doing fine. You say he can't eat normal food. What am I supposed to do?"

"Okay, I'm taking her home tomorrow, and I don't have a clue about how this is all going to work. Don't any of you people worry about that?"

"Nobody ever prepared me for this! Who do they think I am—Einstein?"

---

Another way to approach differences in values is to develop the ability to take another's perspective. The effectiveness of the counseling process often depends on being able to see things as the other sees them. Empathy, for example, is rooted in the ability to shift perspective. Many things we ask clients to do clinically may seem opaque to them, or not clearly related to improving speech, language, hearing, or swallowing. Seeing our tactics through another person's eyes increases our insight into how we may present information.

A final note on this issue is to remind readers to be beware of their stereotyping tendencies, and to be alert for them. Let us assume that we all have stereotypes, some recognized, some hidden from us. When you are confronted by a person whose appearance or behavior catches you in the midst of one of your own stereotypes, learn from it—and enjoy what you learn. One of Audrey's recent experiences in this regard was an encounter with a highly placed official from the FBI, whose talk I was obliged to attend. I expected the speaker to be a seriously rumpled and unstylishly dressed guy, rather blunt, boring, and inarticulate. Instead, she was immaculately groomed, elegantly attired, gave a dynamic talk, and I hated her for her gorgeous high heels. But I also learned about myself, an opportunity never to be missed.

### Are You Sensitive to Cultural Differences?

All therapeutic endeavors occur in cultural contexts; thus, cultural factors demand awareness and sensitivity in our roles as clinicians and counselors. When a clinician fails to understand and accept the cultural values of a particular client and family and, as a result, fails to place various clinical activities within the mores and beliefs of that culture, clinical intervention will be unsuccessful. This is true even when all of the work is done in a spirit of sincere good will and honesty.[1]

Clinicians must take the steps necessary to develop cultural sensitivity that is intrinsic to their success. Some texts that are particularly relevant to multicultural concerns in communication counseling are those by Payne (1997), Goldberg (1997), Wallace (1993), and Battle (2012). A comprehensive bibliography is available at the American Speech-Language-Hearing Association (ASHA) website (http://www.asha.com) through the link entitled "General issues and multicultural populations."

---

[1]For a poignant and instructive example, read Fadiman's remarkable book, *The Spirit Catches You and You Fall Down* (1997), an exploration of a clash of American medical values and those of a family of the Hmong culture.

Understanding a client's culture is critical to successful counseling. Effective counselors learn about the cultural backgrounds of the persons with whom they work, a task that becomes increasingly daunting as society becomes more culturally diverse. At a minimum, effective counselors must respect and accept cultural differences. Value and culture issues are explored in Box 3–7.

---

**Box 3–7. Exercise: When Cultures and Values Clash**

1. Answer the questions for the following scenarios involving a clash of cultures or values:

   ■ A person states: "I am not comfortable with people who are not forthright enough to look me in the eye." Suggest a clinical/cultural encounter that might present problems for this person. If the person is the counselor, how might this expressed attitude affect a clinical interaction? If the person is a client who is the mother of a child with cerebral palsy, what are some possible effects?

   ■ An 85-year-old woman who has just had her third stroke tells you, "Go away! Leave me alone! I don't want speech therapy!" You know that her speech and language are impaired. In addition, you suspect that she has multiple-infarct dementia and may not be thinking clearly. You think you could be of help. What are some value differences between you that may be reflected in her comments and your reactions?

2. Make a list of five of your personal values. For each value, name some individuals or groups of individuals whose corresponding values may differ. For example, a personal value may be stated as follows: "I believe that Western-style speech-language intervention is useful in adult neurogenic communication disorders." By contrast, some Native Americans who believe that individuals who have incurred strokes have been blessed in some special way may question this value.

---

## Are You Optimistic and Positive?

Many disorders that fall within the scope of practice for SLP-As appear to be bleak, and many deal with tragedy. To be effective counselors, SLP-As must remain realistically optimistic and actively seek the positive. Reality, as Schneider points out, is fuzzy, and so is knowledge (Schneider, 2001).[2] Because communication disorders are complex in nature, clinicians and counselors who are technically skilled in working with affected persons and their families also must be affirming and upbeat. This is important not only for helping families and clients to discover ways to "broaden and build," as discussed in Chapter 2, but because clinicians need these qualities to avoid burnout. Clinicians who remain enthusiastic and positive, who are able to look on the bright side, and who are fascinated by complex problems can make a gift of their optimism to the persons with whom they work.

This quality of personal optimism should not be confused with being a "Pollyanna person"—someone who is consistently positive or forcedly cheerful even in circumstances in which such an outlook is unrealistic and therefore inappropriate. Late on a Friday afternoon, Audrey once heard a student clinician say to a client on a respirator in an intensive care unit: "Have a great weekend." This is not recommended.

## Do You Have a Good Sense of Humor?

To many clinicians, emphasizing a sense of humor may seem misplaced. Yet a working ability to see the light side, as well as the bright side, is a vital attribute of the successful counselor. Norman Cousins (1991) noted that laughter was an essential part of his recovery from a life-threatening disease. Simmons-Mackie's delicious bow to humor in aphasia therapy (2004) should be mandatory reading for all clinicians. People who can appreciate humor or even laugh at themselves probably cope better with these often

---

[2]For a more thorough explanation of the complex nature of tricks that our eyes and brains play on us in this regard, see Gilbert's *Stumbling Toward Happiness* (2006).

messy communication disorders than persons who are more somber. Of course, many people (with and without communication disorders) are dour and humorless; however, if their clinicians and counselors have the ability to see the funny side of life, it can help to balance their own perspectives, decrease their burnout, and enliven the experiences of those with whom they work.

## Are You Flexible?

The challenging (and changing) nature of communication disorders requires those clinicians who counsel affected persons and their families to be adaptable and flexible enough to change approaches and goals in the face of new data, whether those data be of a general nature or specific to a particular person. Because of the fluid state of current health care delivery, the ability to operate effectively within the system also demands flexibility.

## Can You See Beyond the Obvious?

It is important for the clinician-counselor to be able to see beyond the obvious—to recognize more subtle psychosocial factors that may affect the counseling process—and to address any relevant problems as appropriate. Difficulties within the client's family relationships or stresses associated with dealing with the communication disorder may impede clinical progress, as in the following example:

> It is not hard to deduce that Tucker probably is going to have a pretty rough day in speech therapy, because he and his mother arrive late and apparently frazzled for today's session with you. In addition, his mother forgot to bring his implant device. Moreover, Tucker's mother asks you the same questions every week and shows virtually no follow-through on any of the plans you have sent home with her, or the advice you have given her. What do the lateness, the forgetfulness, the repetitive questioning, and the lack of follow-through all mean? Are they related? Putting two and two together, you decide that they are: They say "anxious mom"—and an anx-

ious mom can be a real stumbling block to Tucker's success. Her anxiety must be acknowledged and dealt with if Tucker is to thrive.

## Do You Know Yourself? Do You Like Yourself?

Self-respect, self-esteem, and self-knowledge have always been core issues for counselors in any area of counseling. Communication counseling is no different. Self-examination is an ongoing but rewarding process whereby self-acceptance can be achieved. Many approaches to the development of self-acceptance, ranging from formal psychotherapy to disciplined meditation, are recognized. Whichever approach is used, spending time periodically examining one's own life leads to increasing self-acceptance, an important attribute of the successful counselor.

Self-knowledge can be developed in various ways. To begin, communication counselors can look to their own clinical work to uncover clues in this regard. It is helpful to become aware of issues such as the following: "Why am I pleased when this client cancels a session?" "Where does my anger with this client come from?" "Why does a session with this family make me happy?" or "Why do I leave my session with this client feeling sad?" Self-examination on this basis often reveals underlying feelings that, when attended to properly, can clarify some issues regarding not only clients but also ourselves. Remember that your clinician metaphors should be instructive in this regard.

## Do You Like Challenges?

The management of many communication and swallowing disorders is, without doubt, challenging. Such disorders are baffling in their inconsistency and variability. Some entail dealing with end-of-life issues. Communication disorders occur across a spectrum of complex social contexts. They must be treated with little time and even less money, and often in less than ideal environments. For the person who is threatened, rather than energized by challenges, this field may not be suitable.

Some years ago, Audrey asked students in a counseling class to write a brief description of their ideal clients. The next week they each in turn described this mythical person. As the composite morphed in my head, I became quite discouraged. Their ideal client was Mythical Mary Sue, a sweet little 8-year-old girl, dressed to perfection (possibly in pink). Mary Sue did just what the clinician asked her to do, and why not? She had a perfect home life, with parents who did every clinic assignment with their perfectly cooperative and uncomplaining daughter, and she became perfectly cured of her slight phonological problem by the end of the scheduled treatment plan. Halfway through the presentations, I stopped them. "Do you mean this?" I shouted as I summarized perfect little Mythical Mary Sue. "Where's the fun? Where's the challenge? Give little Mary Sue a break! She's so perfect she'll get to be Miss America even if she lisps!"

The class cracked up but got the point. Fortunately, Mary Sue seldom shows up on real clinical caseloads; challenge, not boredom, is much more likely to energize the effective clinician-counselor. Box 3–8 contains a related exercise to help you learn about yourself as a clinician.

## Attitudes

In his famous book, *Man's Search for Meaning* (1989), Victor Frankl describes certain prisoners in concentration camps who spent their days taking care of others in whatever ways they could. He points out:

---

**Box 3–8. Exercise: Personal Attitudes and Client Characteristics: the Ideal Versus the "Nightmare" Client**

1. Write a paragraph or two describing your ideal client. What makes him or her so appealing to you?
2. Now do the opposite: Describe your nightmare client. What characteristics give you problems? Are they yours or those of the client?

---

They may have been few in number, but they offer sufficient proof that everything can be taken from a man but one thing: the last of his freedoms—to choose one's attitude in any given set of circumstances, to choose one's own way. (Frankl, 1989, p. 104)

How we respond to challenge leads directly to a discussion of attitudes. Counselors' attitudes about their roles help to determine the success of their counseling. The following review of attitudes in clinical practice[3] borrows heavily from Webster's (1977) discussion of appropriate attitudes for counselors who work with families of handicapped children.

Particularly critical for communication counselors are the following factors: how one views oneself in relationship to others, how one perceives and handles issues in authority, and, finally, what attitudes one has about the issue of control. Each of these factors is discussed next.

## Relationships with Others

Webster (1977) reminds her readers of Martin Buber's (1958) notion of the "I–Thou and "I–It" dichotomies. When one person approaches another as Thou in a relationship, the other person is respected or even revered. In I–It relationships, the other person is objectified, that is, treated as a subject for analysis. I–It relationships are important for many aspects of interpersonal relationships. For example, it is important to remember and respect others' preferences about many things and to categorize and know facts about others to whom one is close.

But in the I–Thou relationship, the respect (and value) one holds for others is holistic. It is based not on attributes or facts but on an individual's very personhood. Furthermore, I–Thou relationships preclude analysis and dissection and insist on acceptance. In relation to counseling, the I–Thou and the I–It dichotomies permit consideration of questions such as the following: "Is the information I have to offer of greater value to me than the person to whom

---

[3]Development of the ideas that follow has been greatly influenced by Audrey's mentors, Elizabeth Webster and Louise Ward.

I offer it?" "Do I see the persons I counsel as objects to be directed for their own good?" "Do I work with a disorder or with a person?"

A significant example concerns how a clinician chooses to address a client. Many older clients, for example, come from various cultures and mandatory traditions that others be given permission before familiarity can be assumed. Yet it is increasingly and annoyingly common for clinicians, hospital personnel, and other health professionals to assume that first names are perfectly acceptable forms of address. (This may be exceptionally galling when the clinician or staff member is substantially younger than the client addressed.)

This issue is directly related to the I–Thou, I–It dichotomy and its effects on human interaction. It is a simple matter to ask clients how they prefer to be addressed. Clinician-counselors should never make an assumption concerning form of address; rather, they should simply ask what their clients wish to be called. This is an effective way to honor the I–Thou aspect of a clinical interaction and should be practiced by all clinicians and counselors.

## Authority and Locus of Control

The growing voice of the disability movement (e.g., Jordan & Kaiser, 1996) is influencing much of our clinical and counseling work in general. In Chapter 1, the issue of "Who is the expert?" was raised. That notion is revisited here, along with the value of collaborative models, in which individuals, families, and clinicians contribute to shared decision making and treatment planning. Key issues relate to the nature and distribution of authority and the locus of counseling control.

One useful way to examine locus-of-control factors is for skilled counselors to look at themselves in relation to Fromm's (1947) description of "rational versus irrational authority." In Fromm's view, rational authority stems from equality of the so-called authority (in this case, the counselor) and the person with whom this authority is working. Rational authority is related to competence, but authority status is earned, and others must confer it. It is temporary and dependent on changing information and new data, and the authority of others sometimes overrides it. Rational authority-type people admit their mistakes, are not easily threatened, change their minds when new information is presented, and continually seek to improve what they are doing. They treat others as "Thou" rather than "It." Irrational authority-type people, of course, hold different beliefs. They prefer having power over others, have trouble with criticism, admit mistakes slowly, and assume, rather than earn, their authority. Irrational authority types treat others as "It."

Few would like to think of themselves as irrational authority types, but a key feature of rational authority concerns the equality of the counselor and the counseled. Although the counselor has the expertise in the disorder and techniques for its management, the individual and family are specialists and experts in knowledge about themselves. The expertise of counselors lies both in the extent of their general knowledge and in the breadth of their experience with individuals who share certain problems and conditions.

On the other hand, the expertise of individuals and their families resides in the depth of their experience of the disorder and how it manifests for them, that is, they are experts on how a disorder is lived with every day, as well as on what it is like to have the disorder; hence, a consideration of attitudes concerning locus of counseling control progresses naturally from that of I–Thou relationships and rational authority.

It is probably a good idea for clinicians to omit their professional titles when introducing themselves to a client or a family. Fromm's concept of rational authority cautions against the use of titles with clients. For example, Audrey introduces herself to children, parents, partners, and families by saying, "I'm Audrey Holland," rather than "I'm Dr. Holland" (or, worse, "My name is Dr. Holland"). Although this might not always work so well in school settings, for both of us the whole name situation still seems normal. Also we find it averts subsequent wrangling about authority and about how we wish to be perceived. It also permits the freedom to be ourselves and to practice clinical skills in a personally satisfying way without relying on the authority implicit in a title.

The successful communication counselor recognizes the collaborative partnership of clinician, affected person, and family and its dependence on the clinician's attitudes about control in relationship to authority. When clinicians believe that they are the authorities, others involved then become nonspecialists or novices.

Webster (1977) notes:

> Counselors will get along better with parents (and we add, individuals and families) when they understand that whenever one counselor meets with one parent (or one individual with a neurogenic communication disorder, or with his or her family there are two (or more) specialists involved. (p. 67)

Webster goes on to say that perhaps counselors should consider the following question: To what extent do I believe I can solve this problem? She suggests that communication counselors who feel responsible for taking the lead in solving problems are likely to provide copious amounts of advice and to feel successful only when that advice is acted upon. A better alternative involves respecting clients and their families as capable of managing their own lives, clarifying those aspects that need changing, and encouraging clients to carry out their own solutions; thus, a good counselor should be a participant in the counseling process, not its director.

## Technical Skills

What are the basic skills of a good counselor? Numerous authorities list many different skills. Recall from Chapter 1 that Webster and Newhoff (1981) included the importance of *listening* to what others wanted to share, to clarify ideas, attitudes, emotions, beliefs, and to provide information and options for change. As listed in Box 1–1, the essential components of counseling are *understanding, explaining, advising,* and *translating* into action. Notice that these basic skills are presented as verbs. They involve active or intentional processes and in fact constitute the dynamics of the counseling process. By contrast, clinician characteristics are nouns; they are static qualities that provide a background against which the active counseling skills operate. Box 3–9 illustrates the importance of definitive action (as represented by verb forms) in the counseling process. Notice that the skills in the first column are "quieter" than those in the second column, that is, their functions are predominantly supportive in nature, whereas those in the sec-

---

**Box 3–9. Counseling Skills: Quiet Skills and Loud Skills**

"Quiet" Skills

- Listening and understanding, empathizing, clarifying, reflecting
- Disclosing
- Affirming

"Loud" Skills

- Informing and explaining, planning
- Advising
- Teaching
- Being a change artist

---

ond column, the "louder" skills, are more oriented to change and growth. Both types seem to be necessary for competent counseling, and in actual use, their boundaries frequently are blurred.

## The "Quiet" Skills

### Listening and Understanding

Listening has already been discussed. It is important to remember, however, that *active listening* involves more than just ears. It is signaled by posture, good eye contact (at least in Western cultures), and nonverbal behaviors such as head nodding, judicious pausing, and avoiding interruption and overlaps. It is what Luterman (2008) refers to as "deep listening." Indeed, use of body language to look like an attentive listener is a very important part of the listening process. Everyone has experienced instances in which someone asks (usually impatiently), "Are you listening?" or "Do you hear what I am saying?" Those questions usually are triggered not by any evidence of ear malfunction but by what the rest of the body is doing. Although listening is not synonymous with understanding, it certainly is the main requirement.

Clinicians must recognize the importance of getting beyond the words and the syntax not only when we teach language, but when we counsel. *Understanding* clearly is decoding and comprehending, but it also connotes empathy. For example, people may listen to and comprehend what a certain politician says, but they certainly do not empathize and thus do not truly understand the message behind the politician's comments. (They cannot know the specific aspect of personal background or experience, for example, that led to a particular public decision or stated belief.) Counselors must listen with the "third ear," as noted earlier, and in fact attend with something like the Buddhist concept of the *third eye* as well. A problem with understanding is that counselors sometimes presume to understand when in fact they may not. It is crucial to understand in order to help; thus, many of the important counseling skills are simply ways to validate and clarify our understanding.

How do we become better, more understanding listeners? Here are some suggestions:

- Practice *full-body listening*. Incorporate the culturally relevant nonverbal behaviors into listening. For a majority of persons in today's society, these behaviors include the following: leaning forward, using appropriate eye contact, nodding in agreement occasionally, and so on; in effect, *looking* like a listener.
- Ignore distractions to the listening process.
- Do not fidget.
- Try to listen with the "third eye" and "third ear." Listen for disconnect versus consistency between what is being said and the underlying message. Try to empathize.
- For clients whose intelligibility is impaired, help them to buttress their speech with writing, gestures, and other means.
- Use other counseling skills to confirm understanding.

## Empathizing

In advising health care workers how to avoid burnout, Papadatou (1997) suggests that they try to maintain an attitude of "detached concern." This attitude is almost a polar opposite of empathy, and it is difficult to discern how a committed communication counselor can counsel while maintaining detached concern. Many self-help books have been written on how to become more empathic. In a way, the abundance of such books is scary: If this is truly a market-driven economy, then there must be many people who feel they lack empathy. Some writers use the terms "empathy" and "compassion" as synonyms. "Sympathy" also is sometimes included, but it appears connotatively to lie closer to "pity," which is seriously less desirable in interactions with clients. A more useful and appropriate term is "compassion," particularly in relation to counseling, because it implies a desire to be of service to others. Eric J. Cassell, a physician, described his compassion as follows:

> As I hear my patient recount the story of his illness and all its pain and sadness and see the sickness speaking from his features, my compassion is aroused. I become connected to the patient; we have begun to fuse. I am no longer in an ordinary social interaction where the "distance" between the participants is maintained and where attempts to get closer than the particular culture allows may be perceived as a broach of social convention.
>
> When that happens, I begin to listen, look, and intuit with greater intensity, and more information flows toward me. If I make myself conscious of what is happening, I can begin to feel the patient's emotions, and even my hand palpating the abdomen appears to receive more information than it otherwise would. (Cassell, 2005, p. 443)

Even without the palpating hand, Cassell's remarks serve as a model of the compassion, or empathy, for which communication counselors ideally strive. Cassell further notes that compassion is gleaned primarily through years of experience; however, the first step in achieving compassion, or empathy, comes from growing closer to what others are going through.

Experiences in our daily lives can offer empathy lessons. For example, how do you feel when you are too sick to engage in your normal life, or have to miss long-anticipated events? Or when a physician examines you with "detached concern"? Or when people give advice starting with something like, "You know what you should do?" Compare these feelings with those experienced when another person communicates a sense of direct and total concern for your difficulties. Brief trips to the empathy bank do not have to wait solely on time and experience; rather, empathy can be learned from example. Consider the examples provided by the citizens of Lake Providence discussed in Chapter 2, or the national grieving for the bombing victims that followed the 9/11 attacks.

A final note of caution: Empathy moves us along toward a feeling of walking in someone else's shoes, but it is not truly walking in them. Even when you have had an eerily parallel experience to one you are hearing about, resist the urge to say, "I know just how you feel!" In fact, no one can ever know just how another person feels. Empathy still stops short of being in another's skin. You can only know just how *you* feel.

### Clarifying and Reflecting

*Clarifying* is a two-way process, particularly in counseling clients who have communication disorders. In other words, although clarifying originally was meant to cover a group of techniques whereby a counselor helps a person to understand better or to give more precise words to their own ideas and feelings, it also covers ways of making sure that the counselor actually comprehends what the speaker is saying. In both cases, the technique involves careful questioning and restatement. Some clarifying phrases intended to help clients gain self-understanding are, "I think I hear you say that . . . " (and its variants) and "Let me see if I understand: Is this an example?" An especially useful clarifier is the direct request, "Please help me to understand."

The same kinds of clarifications can be used when it is the counselor-clinician's understanding that is of concern. One trick is to shift responsibility for communication failure from the speaker to the counselor. For example, "I'm having a bad listening day" is always useful, or "I'm missing something here . . . can you tell me again?" Compare, "You probably should speak more slowly, since it's not getting through to me," or even "You need to tell me that again." Both of these place the burden of communication on the client and may inhibit his or her openness in communicating.

*Reflecting* usually is a direct application of a Rogerian non-directive therapy technique (Rogers, 1965). Reflecting refers to a strategy whereby the clinician states back to the client, or restates the underlying (latent) content of, the client's messages. It is not an exact replication of the message. For example, a man with significantly impaired speech following a stroke may state: "I am really angry at the way the health care system is jerking me around!" This could be restated as, "You're feeling used by the folks down at BCD," rather than as, "You are feeling really angry." The goal of reflection is to move this client forward in his ability to see his situation with increased clarity; thus, the first response signals encouragement to be more specific about the "jerking around." The second, overly simple restatement is not nearly so likely to elicit any client response beyond "Yes, I am"—or may even precipitate "That's what I just said!" from an angry and frustrated client.

## Disclosing

*Disclosing* is the straightforward act of sharing a bit of oneself with a client. It also entails limiting disclosure to relevant issues, not sharing one's life story with a client. The goal of disclosure is similar to that of clarifying and reflecting, that is, to help the client move along with increased insight into his or her behavior. Statements such as "When my mother was sick, I felt helpless, too," for example, are appropriate forms of disclosure. So are comments that help the client to understand that you have had pertinent experiences, such as, "My grandmother had Parkinson disease, too." This kind of disclosing helps to build empathy.

Clinicians often are warned of the dangers of bringing too much of themselves into clinical interactions, and disclosing is a practice to be followed cautiously. Indeed, it is a fine line to walk, but an important one. Sharing is what conversation is all about, and SLP-As, especially, recognize the importance of conversation in communication. For example, the clinician may choose to work on a topic in an aphasia conversation group such as "my most embarrassing moment." Which of the following approaches would be more likely to get the group involved?

- Approach 1: The clinician announces at the beginning of the session: "Today we are going to discuss our most embarrassing moments. George, think for a minute, and tell us about yours."

■ Approach 2: "Wait till you hear what happened to me this morning when I was coming into the clinic. I think this was my most embarrassing experience ever!"

Approach 1 probably will result in silence. Who would want to take a chance at such self-exposure? Approach 2 differs fundamentally: The group leader has already taken the chance, and the resulting talk is likely to be a variant on "Can you top this?" (and fun, to boot).

### Affirming

*Affirming* is the easiest of the quiet skills. Indeed, much of it is itself quiet. Affirming means communicating what Rogers calls "unconditional positive regard" (Rogers, 1992). According to this notion, the counselor is on the client's side, is there to help, and is there to understand. It is as important for clients as it is for counselors to recognize and celebrate their own strengths if they are to flourish. Affirming also can be verbal, and much of it should be, particularly if direct clinical work focuses on modifying impairment.

The *counseling moments* in subsequent chapters can serve as occasions to practice many of the quiet skills just outlined. Communication counseling frequently is an integral part of any clinical interaction. All of these skills can be improved with practice, and they can be applied not only in clinical situations but also in interactions with family and friends or with a counseling partner. They certainly will not detract from already-in-place "people skills" and in fact should enhance them.

### The "Louder" Skills

Robert Shum, a clinical psychologist with extensive experience in working with families of children with communication disorders, has commented that SLP-As are masters at explaining and informing, but their other counseling skills are not as well developed.[4]

---

[4]Van Riper Lecture, Western Michigan University, 2004.

Our own clinical observations support his view. SLP-As understand their important role in providing facts to families and adults with communication disorders. In some instances, however, information may be presented too early, or it may not be repeated frequently and thus may not be fully understood or useful to the recipients.

Of greater importance, many SLP-As appear to think that informing, advising, and planning are synonymous with counseling. This is not the case. They do pervade the entire clinical process, along with teaching and encouraging change. All of them permeate the rest of the book; however, good clinicians, adept as they are at teaching and establishing new behaviors, often fail to take the difficulty of moving those new behaviors into habitual use. Although we talk about "generalization," few of us are trained in how to effect long-term changes; therefore, in what follows we take a special look at change, and how behavioral change (generalization) comes about.

## Clinicians as Change Artists

Change is hard. But changing something is essentially what we ask clients, or families, to do. We are about the business of change and growth—from learning an accurate /r/ sound or helping parents to promote language in their autistic child to getting an aphasic individual to complete his homework. Providing clinical techniques for acquiring the new /r/, for helping to promote the requisite language skills, for reacquiring once-easily accessed words, or fitting the appropriate hearing aid—these things are what we are really good at doing. Moving their use into daily life is fuzzier, and generalization data are often sparse, or perhaps not even attended to, beyond anecdotal reports and pre-post changes on standardized measures. But moving those new skills and behavior patterns into daily life is where the action is. An appropriately fitted hearing aid that spends its time in the bureau drawer, or the new /r/ sound that reverts to the old one at the clinic exit door means we have not accomplished our tasks, and that clients have not met their goals. It is our opinion that improvements noted on formal pre- and posttraining tests are inadequate for measuring these kinds of long-term change and growth. We believe generalization is a pervasive clinical issue, involving both technical skills of the profession, but more importantly also counseling skills and abilities.

To demonstrate how hard change is, try changing a behavior of your own that bugs you, or that interferes with your personal sense of who your are. A good exercise in our counseling classes is to ask students to choose a behavior that bothers them, or that represents something they would like to learn, and to make a commitment in writing both to themselves and to the instructor to change or to make inroads into learning the new behavior by the end of the term. Importantly, students must also agree to keep a weekly diary about how it is going and hand in the diary and a summary at the end of the term. The diary is useful because our feelings and our intellectualizing about behavior are seldom in sync, and these records aid us in recognizing the asynchrony, typically the result of this clash between our emotional and our thinking selves.

The notion of duality in human enterprises has been around since at least Plato, who talked about the forces that guide us being akin to an elegant team of horses driven by a skilled charioteer who is responsible for controlling them, and determining how their races should be run and won. Freud's id and ego, more recent descriptions of the planner and the implementer, popular oversimplifications of right and left brain, and so forth, all reflect the dichotomy between our thinking (the charioteer) and our emotional selves (that team of horses). A particularly compelling metaphor (here we go again!) of this duality is explicated by Haidt in his book, *The Happiness Hypothesis* (2006). For Haidt, an elephant (the emotional side of things) replaces Plato's horses, and its rider becomes the charioteer (the practical decider, the one who chooses how the elephant should be ridden and where he is going). We prefer Haidt's metaphor, primarily because the emotions are not always elegant and spirited; they are often larger, more plodding, and more mysterious. Riders or charioteers: take your pick. But charioteers have training and even weapons. Most of us just ride.

So what does this have to do with change? The clearest way is by acknowledging the often differing plans of the powerful elephant and its perhaps more focused rider, and to use the strengths of both of them in a positive way. Elephants (and emotions) represent strength and power; riders (and most frontal lobe functions) represent guidance.

Heath and Heath in the thoroughly delightful and easy-to-read book, *Switch* (2010), use Haidt's metaphor to provide a simple template as a way to harness and respect the elephant in the service of the logical guidance of the rider. The book itself is loaded with examples and illustrations of how to effect change, and it serves as a model of change that is easily adaptable to communication disorders. It is not the purpose of the present book to detail it here, but Box 3–10 adapts their template to our professional needs and hopefully whets your interest for further explanation.

---

### Box 3–10. How to Make a Switch

*For things to change, somebody somewhere has to start acting differently.*

Picture that person (a child with a phonological disorder, an aphasic adult who wants to tell the story of who he is, a spouse who needs time alone and does not know how to achieve it).

*Each of us has an Emotional Elephant side and a Rational Rider side.*

The clinician's role is to help the child, the person with the aphasia, or the spouse to reach both sides and to help to clear the way for them to succeed. In short, three things must be done:

1. Direct the Rider

    *Follow the bright spots.* Investigate what is working and clone it (e.g., What are the client's strengths? How can I bring them to bear on his or her problem?)

    *Script the critical moves.* Do not think big picture, think in terms of specific behaviors. (Design some simple steps in the direction of the goal.)

*Point to the destination.* Change is easier when you know where you are going and why it is worth it.

2. Motivate the Elephant

*Find the feeling.* Knowing something is not enough to cause change. Bring in feelings and capitalize on them. (For young children, this might be the excitement of parents when their child says a new word, or uses appropriate, intelligible sounds. For adults, it might be finally using grandkids' names again, or for families, when you finally have an hour alone.)

*Shrink the change.* Break down the change until it no longer spooks the Elephant; not all the /r/ words, just initially a few that count (blessed be the clinician whose client's name is Ricky); just one grandchild consistently named; just a brief trip to the local Starbucks to bring home a cup of coffee.

*Grow your people.* Cultivate a sense of identity and instill the growth mindset. We have taken a step . . . we can do this! This is the power of aphasia groups, for example.

3. Shape the Path

*Tweak the environment. When the situation changes, the behavior changes. So change the situation.* Help families and all relevant parties to set up reinforcing situations.

*Build habits. When behavior is habitual, it is "free" . . . it does not tax the Rider.* Practice, practice, practice—insist on it, require homework, journals, and so forth

*Rally the herd. Behavior is contagious. Help it spread!* Get all involved persons (siblings, other family members, and so forth, aware of what the goals are. Advertise them. Give others helping roles.

---

(Adapted from Heath & Heath, 2010.)

# Conclusion

The *completely* quiet skills have been saved for last. It is one thing to know what to say and when to say it; it is quite another to know when to say nothing at all. Meister Eckhard noted in the fifteenth century that "silence is one of the best ways to view God." Being silent, as well as practicing the judicious benefits of pausing, is critical to effective counseling. Much that is beneficial in counseling occurs during the silences and pauses that signal serious contemplation, careful consideration, and deep reflection. The goal of counseling, after all, is not to fill space with sound, but to fill space with sound interaction.

A number of issues that relate to the personal characteristics of skilled counselors are covered in this chapter, which also reviews personal characteristics and attitudes that may typify successful counselors. The material presented is intended to be suggestive, rather than exhaustive. These issues require ongoing consideration; they recur many times throughout this book.

Box 3–11 presents a deceptively simple exercise that nevertheless provides valuable practice with one of the most important listening tools: silence.

---

**Box 3–11. Exercise: The 30-Second Rule**

Practice the 30-Second Rule for conversation for one week. Anytime someone asks a question, wait 30 seconds before answering. Because the pause is obligatory, the likelihood is that the answer will include reflection, examination of intention, and preview of tone—all things that make for a wiser response.

---

(Adapted from Boorstein, 1997.)

# References

Battle, D. (Ed.). (2012). *Communication disorders in multicultural and international populations* (4th ed.). St. Louis, MO: Mosby.

Boorstein, S. (1997). *It's easier than you think: The Buddhist way to happiness.* New York, NY: Harper Collins.

Buber, M. (1958). *I and thou* (2nd ed.) (R. Smith, Trans.). New York, NY: Scribner.

Campbell, K. C. M. (2006). *Pharmacology and ototoxicity for audiologists.* Clifton Park, NY: Delmar Cenage Learning.

Cassell, E. J. (2005). Compassion. In C. R. Snyder & S. J. Lopez (Eds.), *Handbook of positive psychology* (pp. 434–445). New York, NY: Oxford University Press.

Cousins, N. (1991). *The anatomy of an illness as perceived by the patient.* New York, NY: Bantam, Doubleday.

Fadiman, A. (1997). *The spirit catches you and you fall down.* New York, NY: Farrar, Straus and Giroux.

Frankl, V. (1989). *Man's search for meaning.* New York, NY: Washington Square Press.

Fromm, E. (1947). *Escape from freedom.* New York, NY: Holt.

Gable, S., Reis, H., Impett, E., & Asher, E. (2004). What do you do when things go right? The intrapersonal and interpersonal benefits of sharing good events. *Journal of Personality and Social Psychology, 87,* 228–245.

Gilbert, D. (2006). *Stumbling toward happiness.* New York, NY: Alfred A. Knopf.

Goldberg, S. (1997). *Clinical skills for speech-language pathologists.* San Diego, CA: Singular.

Golper, L. A. (1992). *Sourcebook for medical speech-language pathology.* San Diego, CA: Singular.

Goodwin, C. (Ed.). (2003). Conversational frameworks for the accomplishment of meaning in aphasia. In *Conversation and brain damage* (pp. 90–116). Oxford, UK: Oxford University Press.

Haidt, J. (2006). *The happiness hypothesis: Finding truth in ancient wisdom.* New York, NY: Basic Books.

Heath, C., & Heath, D. (2010). *Switch: How to change things when change is hard.* New York, NY: Broadway Books.

Holland, A. (2012). Counseling around the edges of traditional treatment. In Goldfarb, R. (Ed.)., *Translational speech-language pathology and audiology.* San Diego, CA: Plural.

Johnson, A., & Jacobson, B. (1998). *Medical speech-language pathology: A practitioner's guide.* New York, NY: Thieme.

Jordan, L., & Kaiser, W. (1996). *Aphasia: A social approach*. London, UK: Chapman & Hall.

Kockelmann, E., Elger, C. E., & Helmstaedter, C. (2004). Cognitive profile of topiramate as compared with lamotrigine in epilepsy patients on antiepileptic drug polytherapy: Relationships to blood serum levels and co-medication. *Epilepsy and Behavior, 5*, 716–721.

Luterman, D. (2008). *Counseling persons with communication disorders and their families*. (5th ed.). Austin, TX: Pro-Ed.

Maguire, G. (2000) Impact of antipsychotics on geriatric patients. *Primary Care Companion Journal Clinical Psychiatry, 2*, 166–172.

Papadatou, D. (1997). Training health professionals in caring for dying children and grieving families. *Death Studies, 21*, 575–600.

Payne, J. (1997). *Adult neurogenic language disorders: Assessment and treatment. A comprehensive ethnobiological approach*. San Diego, CA: Singular.

Rao, P. (2006). Emotional intelligence: The sine qua non for a clinical leadership toolbox. *Journal of Communication Disorders, 39*, 310–319.

Reik, T. (1948). *Listening with the third ear*. New York, NY: Noonday Press.

Rogers, C. (1965). *Client-centered therapy*. Boston, MA: Houghton Mifflin.

Rogers, C. (1992). The necessary and sufficient conditions of therapeutic personality change. *Journal of Counseling and Clinical Psychology, 60*, 827–832.

Rogers, S. J. (2004). Developmental regression in autism spectrum disorders. *Mental Retardation and Developmental Disabilities, 10*, 139–143.

Satir, V. (1967). *Conjoint family therapy* (rev. ed.). Palo Alto, CA: Science and Behavior Books.

Schneider, S. (2001, March). Realistic optimism. *American Psychologist*, 250–259.

Simmons-Mackie, N. (2004). Just kidding! Humour and therapy for aphasia. In J. F. Duchan & S. Byng (Eds.), *Challenging aphasia therapies: Broadening the discourse and extending the boundaries*. New York, NY: Psychology Press.

Taylor, B. (2005). Emotional intelligence: A primer for practitioners in human communication disorders. *Seminars in Speech and Language, 2*, 138–148.

Vogel, D., Carter, J., & Carter, P. (1999). *The effects of drugs on communication disorders* (2nd ed.). San Diego, CA: Singular.

Wallace, G. (1993). Adult neurogenic disorders. In D. E. Battle (Ed.), *Communication disorders in multicultural populations*. Boston, MA: Andover Medical.

Webster, E. (1977). *Counseling parents of handicapped children: Guidelines for improving communication*. New York, NY: Grune & Stratton.

Webster, E., & Newhoff, M. (1981). Intervention with families of communicatively impaired adults. In D. S. Beasley & G. A. Davis (Eds.), *Aging: Communication processes and disorders*. New York, NY: Grune & Stratton.

Worrall, L., & Egan, J. (2000, July 4–7). *Learning to use the Internet: An approach for communicatively-disordered adults*. Poster presented at the Asia Pacific Conference of Speech Pathology and Audiology, Gold Coast Australia.

Ylvisaker, M., & Feeney, T. (1998). *Collaborative brain injury intervention*. San Diego, CA: Singular.

## Website

Network Connections of Communication Sciences and Disorders: http://www.mnsu.edu/comdis/kuster2/welcome.html

# Chapter 4

# COMMUNICATION COUNSELING WITH PARENTS OF CHILDREN WITH OR AT RISK FOR DISABILITY

*People can live well with any disability if their nations are just, their communities are decent, and their families are supportive and loving. It is OK to be disabled. Disability is not opposed to happiness and quality of life. Why is it that so many of us parents must wait for our children to teach us this fact?*

—Sue Swenson (2004), mother of a child with a severe developmental disability and Executive Director, The Arc of the United States

## Some Fundamentals and Commonalities

It probably is impossible to imagine the overwhelming sense of difficulty and loss for parents who have just begun the process of acknowledging that their child is not perfect. Few if any children (or parents, for that matter) are perfect. Nonetheless, most parents have harbored such a secret wish. Parents of children born with disabilities, who acquire them during childhood, or who are at risk for them face tremendous problems, as their dreams of a perfect child are threatened, if not shattered. This state involves catastrophe, and the stages of crisis loom large. The first stage is shock that this has happened. Even in the face of family history of disorder, when the mother has undergone prenatal testing, or when the parents are otherwise forewarned that all might not be well, shock is common to all affected parents. Then comes realization, then perhaps denial, and finally, acknowledgment. However, rather than orderly progression from one stage to the next, a more common experience is a mixture of the different stages—perhaps a vacillation between magical thinking directed at the notion that the child has been misdiagnosed (overt denial), that exceptions occur, that cures are just around the corner, or that despite the evidence, all will be well (covert denial). These reactions may occur simultaneously with the negativity inherent in having a "damaged child" and what that may mean, not only for the child but also for parents and siblings, for grandparents, and even for society. Additionally, these stages and reactions may be revisited throughout the life of the child as the parents provide for their child amidst constantly changing life circumstances. Although there is often great overlap in the struggles associated with different disorders of childhood, we recognize that certain syndromes, disorders, or classification systems are quite unique; however, it is beyond the scope of this book to address them all individually. Our hope is that we can speak to the concerns that parents may have and the counseling situations that clinicians may find themselves in when dealing with children who have, or are at risk of having, communication disorders.

This chapter focuses on parents and issues confronting them as they deal with the possibility or reality that their child may have a range of communication problems. By design, the focus here is on counseling parents as they strive to come to terms with their child's struggles and as they go about obtaining the support and services their child needs. The strategies and counseling considerations for clinician-child interactions are presented in the chapters that follow; however, as with the preceding chapters, much of the general concepts and approaches that inform our understanding of how to counsel parents flow out of the characteristics and overall mindset that we have taken with regard to SLP-As adopting a wellness perspective toward counseling in general.

Box 4–1 presents a situation revealing potential emotional struggles even the best parents may experience as they work to obtain the understanding, resources, and support that their child needs. Even though the child in this example was older, issues associated with diagnosis and determining how to move forward were tough.

This mother was so oriented toward addressing problems that successes, however small they may have been, were almost entirely missed. While there exist competing and frequently controversial theoretical and clinical positions for how to conceptualize and treat many disorders of childhood, we believe that communication counselors must embrace the child and his family's strengths and help them to consider how to integrate them into addressing their struggles. In the previous chapters we have proposed that medical models that pathologize clients can frequently get in the way of one's ability to move forward. Many childhood disorders have variable courses that affect both the child and his or her parents.

Gergen (2009, 2001) describes the objectives of traditional counseling as being focused primarily on the mental states of the person being counseled. He argues that focus solely on the individual's mental state may limit potential benefits of therapy. Gergen proposes a shift in counseling to a focus on the creation and maintenance of relationships, or what he terms "relational states." From his perspective, progress in counseling therapy is achieved when those involved create meaningful connections with some individual or group. This view fits nicely with the expertise in communication of SLP-As.

---

### Box 4–1. Counseling Parents: Orienting to Strengths

Read the following scenario. Reflect on similar interactions in your own life. What perspective is necessary to help this parent in this potential counseling moment? What might the clinicians do differently as a part of their intake approach in the future?

During a portion of a recent diagnostic evaluation conducted in a university clinic, the student clinician was completing an initial interview and case history intake portion of the evaluation while the clinical supervisor observed in another room on a video monitor. The student provided the mother with the opportunity to describe in detail the concerns and frustrations both the family and school were having with her 15-year-old son who would later be diagnosed as a fairly high-functioning child with autism. The mother easily described academic areas of failure such as reading, writing, and behavior problems in the classroom. She described his failures in interacting with siblings and neighbors, and pointed out that she and his father considered eliminating all outside sources of interaction. She also noted the child's inability to relate to his parents. A truly bleak and unpleasant scenario was painted. The student clinician did a wonderful job getting examples and making sure she understood the family's complaints. For her part, the mother was composed, careful, and clear as she worked through the interview. From the other room, the supervisor anticipated where, in the final report writing, the student clinician might struggle and came into the room to ask the parent a couple of questions. The supervisor innocently (and certainly without knowing the impact of the line of questioning) asked the mother, "You've provided great information about your son's struggles and have helped us understand why there is such frustration. What would you say are a few of the things your child does well?"

The student clinician and clinical supervisor were stunned when the mother burst into tears. The supervisor, uncertain what prompted such an emotional response, apologetically added, "I mean no disrespect." Yet when the mother regained her composure enough to speak, her response was illuminating. She stated something to the effect of, "I've focused so much on what my son can't do; it just dawned on me that I don't really know what strengths he has."

Furthermore, Stanley Greenspan (2001) noted that for meaningful growth to occur, children must feel they can safely express their feelings to the grown ups who are trying to reassure them. This takes time. Even minimal support, say, for example, just understanding, must come from adults who commit themselves to helping children work through the challenges. Although Greenspan's writing is directed generally to security in children, parents of children at risk for, or with, communication disorders probably have even greater need to feel secure. We professionals often find ourselves in situations where we can help meet these needs. Whether we are working on prevention, diagnosis, or treatment, our success with parents will be heavily influenced by how well we understand them, their motivations, and, most importantly, their child's needs. We have suggested that in every therapeutic interaction the SLP-A is only one of the experts in the room. Both clients and parents have much more knowledge and understanding of what it is like to live with the communication struggles themselves.

Both Gergen and Greenspan are suggesting that we must see counseling opportunities as a collaborative endeavor in relationship building where all those involved negotiate to arrive at a shared understanding of the situation. This is how the empowerment needed to move forward is constructed. Toward this aim, we continue to adopt a wellness perspective as we discuss consequences of diagnostic labels and parents' reactions them, the importance of knowing families, as well as strategies for learning their story, their concerns, how to negotiate the system, and how to advocate for their needs.

## Counseling Consequences of Labeling

Parents rarely seek out SLP-As without assuming that a problem may exist in their child's communication abilities. Although SLP-As are not typically the ones who break the news to families that their child has a specific impairment, we are often involved in the process of making diagnosis. Labeling itself can have positive and negative consequences. Without question, SLP-As witness and experience parents' reactions to the impact of labels. These reactions may be immediate or delayed, and can also change over time as the meaning sinks in or as behavior changes.

Labels allow us the opportunity to conceptualize, and discuss symptoms and complaints in an organized manner (Balint, 1957; Damico, Muller, & Ball, 2010). Such clarity and enlightenment is why pursuing a label may be important. Parents may sense that something is amiss and want to know why. They may wonder if it was something they did or did not do that led to their child's struggle. This drive to name the problem may function as a catalyst for parents beginning to move forward and provide more appropriately for their child (Damico & Augustine, 1995). In addition to facilitating understanding, Gillman, Heyman, and Swain (2000) suggest that labels can create opportunities for resources and support that may otherwise be unavailable. We know that appropriately applied labels, in many instances, can direct clinicians and educators to tailor instruction and remediation to more effectively meet the needs of the child and family. Parents and children may also find that the label legitimizes their concerns or enhances self-understanding. One's identity and self-worth, as well as a sense community, can also emerge (Kelly & Norwich, 2004).

Despite these and other potential benefits, the process of labeling can create many counseling moments, that is, there are also potential negative, stigmatizing consequences of the diagnosis (Goffman, 1964; Heise, 2007; Kroska & Harkness, 2008). The process of labeling a communication disorder localizes the problems within the child and in some instances within the family. From appropriately identified communication impairment associated with genetic disorders or acquired injuries, to inaccurately labeled sources of impairment, such as Kanner's "refrigerator mothers" as the cause of autism (Grinker, 2007) or mistaking "speech and language differences" for "speech and language disorders" (Caesar & Kohler, 2007), localizing deficits within an individual may limit the acknowledgement of other influencing factors and extraneous variables (Damico et al., 2010). Counseling moments can arise from frustration associated with a perceived ignoring of the consequence of teaching styles, cultural and linguistic bias or expectations, differences in background experiences, and the impact of poverty on development in the lives of the children. Furthermore, when labels are applied, expectations often change, with the result of modifying opportunities for growth (Connor, 2006; Connor & Ferri, 2005; Hamayan, Marler, Sanchez-Lopez, & Damico, 2013).

Labels for communication disorders are primarily deficit based, that is, they are assigned based on what the child cannot do; thus, noticing and acknowledging personal strengths may be challenging, as alluded to in the scenario described in Box 4–1. As we have claimed earlier, communication counselors can be more responsive if they recognize and use strengths to lessen their client's struggles.

It would be a mistake for clinicians to assume that parents are going to react in a predetermined manner to the consequences of a label. Counseling parents of children with or at risk for communication disorders requires understanding their personal reactions to the impact the label has on their life and helping them recognize strengths and how that which is working can be accentuated; however, an orientation toward wellness can only be achieved if we truly know the parents.

## Reactions to Labeling

Three commonalities associated with reactions to the consequences of diagnostic labels are briefly discussed next. Specifically we consider the shock factor, the chronic factor, and the allocation of resources factor.

## The Shock Factor

Even parents who have been "prepared" by prenatal counseling, have long suspected problems, or have identified and labeled the problem long ago may experience shock upon seeing their own child is different from other children. For many parents, there may be initial shock at seeing one's own child with a craniofacial anomaly, or of finding out that motor development is likely to be slower or different from the normal for their baby with cerebral palsy. Similarly, parents of an adolescent with a pragmatic impairment, such as Asperger syndrome, may also feel a sense of shock when they see their child's social awkwardness in relationship to other children. Our experience has been that parents during these moments are often not ready to absorb information and move forward. This can be a time of catastrophe, and counselors must be sensitive to the importance and power of grieving. Although the time it will take may vary considerably, communication counselors must be alert to appreciate and capitalize on moments when parents are able to process information, suggestions, and so forth. Some problems require direct clinical attention in the earliest phases (for example, adaptations that are necessary for providing adequate nutrition), whereas others may require patience in trusting ongoing intervention. All problems require the sensitivity that permits counselors to be good and patient listeners as parents grieve, as well as to assist them in acquiring the information and confidence that permits them to provide the support their child needs.

## The Chronic Factor

For the disorders that come to the clinical attention of SLP-As, both parent counseling and other professional involvement may fluctuate over the course of childhood. For some problems, other specialists assume the burden of helping parents to manage the issue of the chronic conditions that affect their child and, by extension, their family. Because of the nature of the services we provide, usually by the time SLP-As become intensely involved, chronicity is recognized, if not accepted. Nevertheless, we must be constantly alert to the reality of the lifespan problems many children face, the new hurdles that they will encounter as they mature and the reactions that parents might have to these changes. It is never prudent to predict outcomes, and communication counselors can always use practice responding with at least 100 variants of "I can't predict." In this regard, it is wise to remember that even a clear statement of uncertainty is much more satisfying than no answer at all. Nevertheless, we must not avoid the issue of chronicity, but use the counseling process to help families face each new hurdle with realistic optimism and resilience.

## Allocation of Resources Factor

Poverty in relationship to counseling is described later; however, as the consequences of labeling emerge and evolve, parents and families must decide how they will allocate their resources to address the impact of the disorder. "Resources" as used here goes beyond monetary considerations to include time and emotional expenses as well. Even for the small percentage of individuals with unlimited funds, they also have only a finite number of hours in the day available for the required emotional costs of caring and decision making. SLP-As often can help parents weigh where and how they should allocate money, time, as well as emotional and physical energy to achieve results to meet the family's needs. Communication counselors who have a wellness perspective should be aware of their influence on parents and assist them in making informed decisions. This means looking beyond speech-language-hearing services and recognizing that often the resources spent with us usually represents only a fraction of that which pulls upon the family. For example, Dudley-Marling (2000) describes many challenges that families are presented with when homework is assigned to children who struggle. Time spent on that child's homework might mean spending less time with other siblings or engaging in activities that provide relief from stress. Although not intending to disparage homework or the importance of working on problems, Dudley-Marling notes that teachers (and we could include clinicians) are often unaware of the strain even the "simplest" requirements can create for the family. We have often been frustrated when we have asked families to engage in some task we believed would help the child make progress only to discover that it was not completed. Yet being more strengths oriented and counseling minded might assist us in creating and fostering understanding of the strain placed upon parents' and family's resources.

## The Importance of Stories in Counseling Families

The importance of listening to stories probably is never greater in communication counseling than when the stories concern children. As noted earlier, SLPs are seldom the individuals who break the news to families, although audiologists may not get off so easily. In some ways, this suggests that the limited contact that audiologists may have with deaf or hard-of-hearing children places an extraordinary demand on their counseling skills. Nevertheless, the crucial point is that getting the facts (as in interviewing) or giving the facts (as in providing information) is never enough. Effective counselors who listen to their clients' stories have access to a different, additional database. Indeed, we would argue that truly effectively counselors must understand the situation from the perspective of those involved. Communication counselors listen with an ear to interweaving the stories they hear with planning next steps and ensuring that parents and clinicians understand one another. They are expert at employing strategies to discover the stories of their clients. They use the stories to help them to get comfortably on the other side of the counseling table and as a result build their own compassion and empathy. Listening to stories, and understanding what they mean to the storyteller, are a major way to begin the process of sharing expertise. Parr, Byng, Gilpin, and Ireland (1997) call such stories "the insider view." Stories are a primary data source in much of the diagnostic and vital for counseling. For counseling from a wellness perspective, they are as important as data culled from tests and/or other diagnostic procedures. Stories allow us insight into the lived experiences of those experiencing and living with the disorders.

How does one get stories from parents? Although the process lacks the romanticism of journalism, it lacks none of the pleasures. A 2005 interview on National Public Radio (NPR) with Seymour Hersh is revealing. Hersh is the renowned journalist who revealed the 1968 My Lai Massacre in Vietnam and, more recently (along with CBS), unveiled the tortures at Abu-Ghraib prison (2004). The interviewer asked Hersh how difficult it was to get credible sources to open up to him, particularly given his reputation as a muckraker. He laughed and replied, "Americans love to talk about what they know, and they are amazingly eager and responsive to being asked."

Comments such as this should encourage communication counselors to "just ask." SLP-As can use directives such as, "Tell me your story" or "What's been going on?" or "It would really help me if I knew your story—what you felt and what you were thinking, and that kind of stuff." More formally, SLP-As have borrowed from the field of anthropology and sociology methods for eliciting the stories of those they serve in the form of ethnographic interviews (Damico & Simmons-Mackie, 2003; Simmons-Mackie & Damico, 2003; Spradley, 1979; Westby, 1990).

Ethnographic interviewing techniques, in the form of semi-structured interviews aim to provide insight into perceptions and worldviews of the parent. Westby (1990) describes the process as one where rapport is established so that the appropriate questions are asked of the right people in a way that encourages them to talk about their situations. Efforts are made to minimize the power differential that may inherently exist between clinician and parent. As we conveyed in the previous chapter, to empathize with parents we must be willing to relinquish, to some extent, the locus of control and see the world as they experience it. Predetermined questions may serve as a starting point, but responsiveness to what parents share within the context of these unstructured interviews is what ultimately allows us to understand their concerns and perspectives. Counseling moments arise out of contexts where specific concerns, joys, reactions, or needs are raised. Consequently, a defining characteristic of ethnographic interviewing requires communication counselors to become a student and discover what is relevant, in the moment, from the parent's perspective. Clinicians do well to remember that in these interactions parents are indeed the experts on how they think and feel. To this end, counselors ask carefully worded, open-ended, descriptive questions, allowing the parent to convey their thoughts and feelings about what is of greatest importance. Effective strategies for increasing our understanding of the parent's story include helping them to recount examples and illustrations of their experience. This will help us to understand their language as they use it (Spradley, 1979; Westby, 1990). For example, the father comments, "Ben is always so cranky in the morning." The communication counselors must be aware that their interpretation of "cranky" may differ from that of the father; therefore, it would be useful to ask, "Can you describe for me exactly what happened the last time Ben was 'cranky' in the morning?" Hearing the description contextualized in a real event also assists in interpreting the event's impact on the parent's daily life. Box 4–2 contains some additional helpful hints for getting stories. Adopting the role of a student seeking insight from a parent during such interviews may challenge how the SLP-A sees the situation. The SLP-A and/or the parent's perspective may not be entirely accurate; however, in order for productive counseling moments to unfold, shared understanding is required. When parents feel judged or pressured, our effectiveness as counselors is minimized.

---

**Box 4–2. The SLP-A as Correspondent:
Helpful Hints for Getting the Stories**

- "Help me to understand . . . "
- "What's been happening?
- "If I'm gonna help you, I need to know what's going on."
- "What's the story?"
- "You said you had some news. Tell me all about it."
- "How would you describe a typical homework session with James?"
- "Tell me about the last time you experienced frustration with eating."

---

## What Stories Do

Beyond merely assisting the clinician in understanding the parent's perspective and building relationships of trust, their stories also affect the storyteller. A primary basis for talk therapies in counseling is that through organizing and expressing experiences to others, a narrative also provides an opportunity for reflection, solutions, and acceptance, especially in a safe listening environment (Gergen, 2001, 2008, 2009; Sharry, 2004). Telling their story is one way for parents to become more accepting of, perhaps even comfortable with, what has happened to them. Stories repeated often and over time become ways to grow toward acknowledgment. We cannot and need not solve all of the problems our clients experience. But in the telling of stories, parents might reveal to themselves transparent meanings and clear solutions to problems. SLP-As must resist the urge to impose their own values onto the parents and families; rather, our role is simply to assist parents and families. Often, resolutions to challenges are more meaningful and lasting when they are discovered by the parent rather than forced upon them by a service provider. Being asked and encouraged to relate one's story can facilitate these experiences.

When stories are shared with others, particularly others whose basic stories are similar, they can become mechanisms for personal growth. Stories can be especially potent when levels of perceived catastrophe are made explicit. When a particularly fragile parent hears a more resilient one describe her own successful coping, the fragile parent may find a role model for growth and resilience.

To this end, parent groups provide a fertile ground for such growth among their members. Communication counselors who hear family stories, who remember the stories of others, and who know the power of such disclosure also can be effective in helping parents who are unable to participate in groups. In such cases, the clinician serves as the "surrogate mouthpiece" for many other people, including those whose experiences are documented in books and testimonials. A clinician with a sharp memory and a well-honed bibliography is a rich resource for families. This underscores the necessity of keeping up to date in the search for good stories, books, or films to share.

Far more frequently than specific sessions set aside to talk it over, or to furnish information, counseling moments provide communication counselors with excellent opportunities to be of help to parents. To take advantage of them, the counselor must first be on the lookout for their appearance, and then be responsive to them. Sometimes a question concerning a relatively less important question may signal the presence of a much bigger issue, whereas at other times such questions may indicate the need for simple reassurance. For example, the time management issue is universal and for some parents can be addressed with joint problem-solving work. For others, the time management question may be a way to discover whether they are adequate parents. (This is just a reminder to stay alert for latent content.) Box 4–3 contains some examples of questions from parents about issues that may or may not fall within the SLP-A's scope of practice. A useful way to practice management of counseling moments is to keep a small notebook with you during your days in the clinic. As such moments occur, not only to you but also to your colleagues, jot them down along with their consequences. Then spend time later evaluating how effective the interchanges were and how they might have been improved.

---

**Box 4–3. Exercise: Scope-of-Practice Boundaries with Specific Clinical Scenarios**

The following comments from parents of at-risk infants and toddlers each define a specific clinical scenario. As the clinician in each case, decide whether the resulting "counseling moment" is within your scope of practice. If it is not, then answer from that perspective. If you decide it is within your scope of practice, answer from that perspective. Try for more than one answer. Feel free to add relevant context.

"How can you discipline a 2-year-old who doesn't understand you?"

"She takes up so much of my time and energy that I'm close to ignoring my other kids."

"We really can't decide on the pros and cons of a cochlear implant for Louie. What should we do?"

"I wish I could figure it out. Nothing like this ever happened to me before. I don't think I can manage this teenager!"

"We just found out the most amazing thing! They've found that there is a link between eating bananas and autism. We have already stopped eating them, and I think I can see a difference in Frances already! What do you think?"

"I really am a nervous wreck. I lie awake and worry if he's even getting enough to eat, and every time he cries, I just go all to pieces."

"What am I to do? He cries every morning on the way to school and has trouble falling asleep on school nights."

"Can you help us think of something to do that might help my wife and me to feel a little better about ourselves?"

"If I have to remind Tom once more to pay some attention to his little brother, I think I'll scream. Tom would be better with him if Teddy didn't have cerebral palsy, I feel sure."

"Am I really an okay mom? How do other parents do it?"

"My wife Suzy thinks this problem is with the genes on my side of the family, and I'm to blame. I wish I knew how to deal with that."

# Issues of Concern to Parents and Families

## Am I a "Good Parent"?

Most clinicians probably make some implicit assumptions about what it means to be a "good parent." These assumptions are largely constructed as a result of our lived experience or may be based on our own mothers or fathers, or those of friends or individuals who significantly influenced our worldview. This composite is the "good parent" whom we would aspire to be. Not surprisingly, most parents we work with also have implicit assumptions and aspirations concerning themselves as parents. How those aspirations are framed may differ, but they help us to understand the various faces of parenting.

Parents of children at risk for or with communication disorders also have "good parent" aspirations for themselves. Most likely, what they envisioned prior to having a child is different from the reality. When the general challenges of parenthood collide with the unique experience of having a child with a disorder, it is common for parents to wonder if they are a "good parent." This nebulous attribute can haunt parents as what they thought would be is confronted with what is. We must be careful that our definition of what constitutes a "good parent" does not infringe upon that of the parents we serve. Values vary substantially and yet no one view is right or wrong—views are just different. Finding out what good parenting means to a mother or father is basic to providing appropriate counseling. It is important for the clinician-counselor to refrain from trying to change values; rather, all values should be respected. One aspect of parent counseling is to help parents to understand their own aspirations, to follow their own dreams, and to make appropriate modifications when their child differs from their expectations. The "child who might have been" is possibly a ghost in the treatment room.

This idea of a ghost, present but not visible, comes from an influential parenting essay by Fraiberg, Adlson, and Shapiro: "Ghosts in the Nursery" (1975). The ghosts in this essay are one's own parents and their often unrecognized and unseen influences on an individual's parenting styles. But there may be others, such as the "child who might have been" just mentioned. How does the communication counselor find out which ghosts are affecting parents? Of course, knowing and understanding parents' stories and being skilled at getting them to share their experiences is one way we have already described. Another way is by carefully observing the interactions between parents and their child and giving careful attention to the things they attend to most. The unspoken "tells" of parents can reveal priorities that may or may not be realized. Where appropriate, a communication counselor can help parents discover these values so that the question of what a "good parent" is can be defined by the values they hold and are comfortable with, by observing and listening intently, by questioning, restating, confirming, and so forth, the concern of quality.

## Will She/He Ever . . .

"Will my child ever go to college?" "Will she ever marry?" "Will he ever be able to read on grade level?" "Will she ever talk?" "Will he ever make friends like other children?" "What will happen to her when I'm gone?" These and similar "What will" questions are often what cause parents to lie awake at night and what can prompt many of the counseling moments we experience. One of the advantages of working with children is that their futures typically hold promise and surprise, and unfortunately, even shock beyond what can be imagined today.[1]

Some diagnoses are disintegrative or degenerative; however, for most disorders of childhood, development greatly enhances the potential for improvement. While SLP-As certainly do not have crystal balls that illuminate the future of children with communication disorders, parents often ask us our thoughts on what the future holds for their child. We believe that this is a quite natural question and one that needs to be valued and honestly addressed. We know that typically the more pervasive and profound the level of impairment, the more likely it is that the disorder will affect a child throughout his or her life; however, many times we simply do not know for certain. Some years ago, right after the first edition of this

---

[1]For a comprehensive, positive, and often unsettling exploration of the potential differences between parents and children, scholarly clinicians are urged to explore "Far from the Tree" (Solomon, 2012).

book, Ryan enrolled in Audrey's graduate course in counseling. On the first night of class, Audrey taught two very critical counseling techniques that every SLP-A must learn. The first technique is to not be afraid to say, "I don't know." The second technique makes an excellent chaser: "But I'll do my best to help you find out." Willingness to acknowledge limitations in our knowledge base while reaffirming our commitment to the family and child is much better than providing misleading or incorrect information. Furthermore, simply dismissing the question without considering why it is being asked at that time fails to recognize a potentially important concern.

It is always helpful to have long-range plans and to prepare for major transitional stages like entrance into preschool, elementary, middle, and high school. Also, parents need to prepare for transitions from their child's school-aged years into adulthood and what will happen when the parents are no longer around or able to provide for their child. The aspirations and dreams parents have for their children should be considered and worked toward; however, the day-to-day obsession with events in the distant future should not prevent working toward the goals that are realistically obtainable. It can be very damaging for parent and child for clinicians to dismiss these dreams.

Communication counselors rely on their own understanding of the normal language acquisition process to guide and help parents understand what is going on with their children. Clinicians must be able to convey this information to parents in terms they can relate to, and in the context of their child's concerns. This is an important counseling responsibility, but it should be supplemented with readable, lay-oriented material about normal language as well.

## How Can I Help My Child Find Acceptance?

We have discussed the challenge to the dreams and aspirations that parents of children with communication disorders and frequently accompanying problems experience. As the impact and consequences of a child's communication disorder changes, a parent's goals and objectives may change also. Many parents of children with autism go from wanting a normal childhood to just wanting their child to say something or feel a sense of emotional regulation. Others see their goals of academic success turn into just hoping that their child will find or make one friend. Dudley-Marling (2000) describes his changing goals for his daughter and his wish for her to be somewhere safe from both the perceived and real ridicule by bullies. Unfortunately, children with communication disorders are frequently perfect targets for bullying and too often experience subtractive environments where their strengths are not valued (Heinrichs, 2003; Laminack & Wadsworth, 2012). In these circumstances, communication counselors must be sensitive to changes and willing to shift focus to meet the family's potentially evolving needs.

## Negotiation and Advocacy within the Systems

We are consistently confronted by parents and caregivers exasperated with the systems governing resources and access to services. Even parents who have had a child receiving services may experience bureaucratically induced frustration or even uncertainty as a child changes schools, as clinicians and teachers change from year to year, as insurance coverage evolves (or in some cases devolves), and as the laws and application of laws changes within school districts and other institutional programs. Given today's political climate and economic struggles, it is easy to become cynical about state and private education systems and insurance companies. Yet communication counselors need to be able to step up and assist parents of children with or at risk for communication disorders as they navigate and negotiate whatever system with which a specific parent might be dealing.

We assume that usually service providers associated with families like the one described in Box 4–4 are moving within the parameters of the law and undoubtedly doing their best to manage large and hectic caseloads. Typically, teachers are motivated to help where they can as well. Understanding the parent's frustration and recognizing the challenges of working with and within the system allows SLP-As opportunities to work together to come up with potential options. Some options, like those described in the case example, may merely function as bandages and attempts to hold on until professional services can be obtained, others may include strategies for how to work with the child. Additional resources may include efforts to assist in better navigating the system. All of the

**Box 4–4. Negotiating Systems**

This story contains elements of what we believe SLP-A communication counselors should be able to address:

> A few years ago, Ryan sat in a session with a parent to present evaluation findings about a second grade child desperately in need of support and intervention with literacy acquisition. After learning that her child would have to be placed on a waiting list to receive services at the university clinic, the mother explained that her finances were limited and that the school system was in the process of qualifying her daughter for services. She was glad that the recently completed evaluation provided clear and convincing evidence regarding the type of support that might help address the issues. Yet, in exasperation the mother turned to Ryan and said something to the effect of, "I get it that my daughter needs help. What am I supposed to do while I wait for her to qualify or for a slot to open up? By the time that happens the school year will be half over and she'll just be further behind!"

What this parent needed was not a smug academic making points she already understood; rather, she needed help developing strategies for navigating the system and accessing the resources that would meet her child's needs right now. Consequently, Ryan provided the mother with easy-to-understand books and materials, written for parents, on understanding literacy development. Box 4–5 provides a list of resources. In this case, Smith's *Book of Learning and Forgetting* (1998) and Trelease's *Read Aloud Handbook* (2006) were recommended to the mother. Additionally, to make access to these resources easier, copies of the books were located and corresponding card catalog call numbers from the library in the family's community were provided. These resources were intended to help the mother become more informed about how learning to read occurs and some roles she could take in the process. Lists of appropriate and enjoyable children's books were provided, again with references to where they could be found. Websites were provided in writing as well as via hyperlinks in an e-mail to sites relevant to the interests and needs of the child and family (see Internet addresses listed at the end of the chapter for ideas). These resources were provided to the mother because they contained books, and activities geared to her daughter's interests. The intent was that such resources would both help the child learn to read and, perhaps more importantly, provide opportunities for enjoyable interactions for the family. YouTube clips were shared demonstrating some of the strategies appropriate for the parent. To address issues of navigating the system, names of families in the community who had experienced and successfully negotiated their way through similar frustrations and had agreed to share their experience were provided. With the mother's permission, Ryan passed along her contact information to these families.

strategies should empower the family with information and options so that they can have some increased measure of control over the situation while minimizing, to the extent possible, some of the barriers to accessing these resources. Communication counselors must recognize opportunities for counseling in these settings and must be informed enough to guide parents to answers that work for them. As in the case above, some families may not have access to the ideal, so those involved must do the best they can with the resources available. We now discuss a few of them, namely, what communication counselors must know, what the accompanying problems are, and how can communication counselors advocate.

## What Must Practicing SLP-A Communication Counselors Know?

The most effective communication counselors rely on their own understanding of the normal language acquisition process to guide and help parents understand what is going on with their children.

---

**Box 4–5. Books on Language Acquisition**

Acredolo, L., & Goodwin, S. (2002). *Baby signs: How to talk with your baby before your baby can talk to you.* Lincolnwood, IL: NTC Publishing.

Apel, K., & Masterson, J. J. (2001). *Beyond baby talk: From sounds to sentences. A parent's complete guide to language development.* Roseville, CA: Prima Publishing.

Fox, J. (2008). *Your child's strengths: Discover them, develop them, use them: A guide for parents and teachers.* New York, NY: Viking/Penguin Press.

Golinkoff, R. M., & Hirsh-Pasek, K. (1999). *How babies talk: The magic and mystery of language in the first three years.* New York, NY: Dutton/Penguin Press.

Greenspan, S. I. (2002). *The secure child: Helping our children feel safe and confident in a changing world.* Cambridge, MA: First Da Capo Press.

Hirsh-Pasek, K., & Golinkoff, R. M. (2003). *Einstein never used flash cards: How our children really learn and why they need to play more and memorize less.* Emmaus, PA: Rodale Press.

Kohn, A. (2005). *Unconditional parenting: Moving from rewards and punishments to love and reason.* New York, NY: Atria Books

Lareau, A. (2011). *Unequal childhoods: Class, race, and family life* (2nd ed.). Berkley, CA: University of California Press.

Perlstein, L. (2003). *Not much just chillin': The hidden lives of middle schoolers.* New York, NY: Random House.

Smith, F. (1998). *The book of learning and forgetting.* New York, NY: Teachers College Press.

---

We see this is an important counseling responsibility, but it should be supplemented with readable, lay-oriented material about normal language as well (see Box 4–5 for some suggestions). The mother we described in Box 4–4 was provided with a number of resources that could be developed based on where she was in her understanding of language and literacy acquisition. Specific facts about the disorders we work with can have powerful influences on communication counseling. It is inappropriate here to review the full breadth of knowledge that affects the counseling process, because such knowledge, both of the disorders and of their specific interventions, has been basic to formal coursework in the study of human communication and its disorders.

A primary responsibility of clinician-counselors in any job is to augment their knowledge with as much relevant information as possible. This information should come from a number of sources: books, colleagues, videotapes, websites, parents, and community resources. It is important to be up to date on professional resources, as well as to know the more general literature or websites that parents are familiar with or that can be recommended. This information, of course, applies fundamentally to the evaluation and treatment of a specific disorder, but a substantial amount of it applies to the counseling aspects of the disorders as well.

The following is an example of some of the essential questions for which parents of children on an SLP-As caseload may need answers. The communication counselor's skill in addressing these types of issues can go a long way toward empowering parents.

1. What are the genetic characteristics of Disorder A?
   - If the parents have other children, are they likely to have this disorder?
   - If they have other children who do not have this disorder, why not?
   - What are the risks for their children as future parents?
2. If it is not a genetics issue, then what is it?
   - Did I [the mother] fail to take care of some aspect of my health? Did I do something wrong?
   - Are we being punished for past misdeeds?
   - Did it just happen? How satisfying is such an explanation?
3. What is the developmental course of Disorder A?
   - What future problems can be foreseen?
   - What potential problems can be forestalled?
   - What does the future hold?
   - Do other problems accompany the communication disorder? If so, what are they?
4. Where is help to be found?
5. What about support groups?

6. What other options are there for treatment?
7. How can I determine which treatments are helpful and which ones are potential scams?

This is only a sampling of relevant questions. They are not meant to encourage communication counselors to overstep the American Speech-Language-Hearing Association (ASHA) Scope of Practice and pretend to be medical experts or genetic counselors, or early childhood education specialists. Rather, they underscore the need for communication counselors to have up-to-date information and an ability to clarify or to repeat what the real experts have said. They also illustrate the tremendous advantage that accrues when SLP-As collaborate with specialists from other disciplines.

It also is important to listen for when parents have misunderstood. In such instances, we can help by referring parents back to the appropriate information sources for clarification and further explanation. To be an effective broker of such information, astute counselors need as much information about parental beliefs as possible, as well as the facts. It is important to recognize that such beliefs often are culturally influenced and may vary widely.

## What About the Accompanying Problems?

Schools of clinician training usually do a sound job of preparing clinicians for preventing, diagnosing, and intervening with children with impairment. Accrediting bodies help see to that and hold aloft standards to serve as guides for clinician education. Furthermore, ASHA makes available a host of resources, position statements, and continuing education opportunities for SLP-As to stay knowledgeable on the causes and changes in assessment and intervention best practices. We have found, though, that knowing how to deal with these types of concerns from parents can take the form of accompanying *alongside problems* for the clinicians. Often these alongside problems are the most daunting.

Let us illustrate what we mean by accompanying problems. Audrey asked a graduate class in counseling to describe their most nightmarish client. She expected them to discuss individuals with communication disorders, such as an adult with primary progressive aphasia, or perhaps an adolescent who stutters. Instead, the students, to a person, described their nightmare clients not by their communication disorders or their age, but by their "alongside problems."

Alongside problems are not the expected cognitive or behavioral concomitants of many of the disorders, such as cognitive or pragmatic problems, or attention deficit disorder, or even sensory and motor accompaniments. Students rightly noted that they had been well prepared through their coursework for those things. Instead, they described problems that fell into two general categories: (1) unwieldy emotional responses in clients and (2) interpersonal issues with their clients' parents. Stillman, Snow, and Warren (1999) described reactions of graduate student clinicians working with children with pervasive developmental disorders and the anxiousness that these alongside problems can induce. Such problems tend to tax our counseling skills, perhaps because they present situations in which clinicians may feel that they are ineffective and inadequate as a result of their lack of training in managing them. Solutions relate to counseling skills.

Many alongside problems also embody parents' anxiety, confusion, and bewilderment about raising children with disabilities. They may concern issues in behavior management, realized in possibly unspoken questions such as, "How can I guide Sean in appropriate behavior when he can't understand me?" or "Who could possibly discipline Nina, with all her physical disabilities?" (See Box 4–6 for some of similar concerns.)

Related alongside issues also may include the extent of trust that parents feel they can confidently place in clinicians who have a large number of children on their caseloads. For example, do Maria's parents trust her clinician to be sensitive to their daughter's special needs? After all, Maria is at the very center of her parents' maelstrom and perhaps represents only a ripple in the water for her clinician. Another parent may wonder, "How can I be sure that any clinician will understand Josh's needs if I am not there to interpret? After all, he has a communication problem."

Sadness and sense of loss frequently accompany the unexpected presence and the challenges of providing for a handicapped child. This may not only produce bewilderment but also can result in parental depression. With depression, the ability to parent effec-

---

**Box 4–6. Parents' Worries for Managing
Life with Their Affected Child**

The following questions may present as accompanying or "alongside" problems. Reflect on what might be the underlying issue. Practice verbalizing how, as a communication counselor, you would respond.

"Do you think I'm a good parent to this child?"

"How do I manage my time?"

"How do I discipline a child with this type of disorder?"

"How should I explain him to others?"

"How do I avoid playing favorites with my other kids?"

"What about our other kids?"

"Where can I get advice for the day-to-day stuff?"

"What about me?"

---

tively is likely to be compromised. This impairment may affect both children with disabilities and their nonhandicapped siblings. Maintaining alertness to depression and anxiety is a constant responsibility of SLP-As.

Finally, there is frequently a cross-cultural component to parental trust. If cross-cultural issues appear to be adversely influencing the counseling relationship, it is imperative that the counselor take the initiative for resolving them, whether by referral, by attempts at open discussion, or by seeking additional help.

SLP-As are not expected to be parenting specialists. Nevertheless, they must be extremely sensitive to such general issues if they are to be effective clinicians. SLP-As must be strong enough to point out children's inappropriate behaviors to parents, particularly if those behaviors have a negative effect on clinical interaction and outcome. Furthermore, if clinicians see parental behavior as the root of their child's problem behavior, they must deal with this as well.

**Box 4–7. Addressing Alongside Concerns**

To develop the ability to address these issues, clinicians can incorporate several practices into their interactions with parents. Reflect on how effective you are at the following:

1. Adopting the initial assumption that parents are doing the very best they can with what they have. (Nobody wants to be a lousy parent.)
2. Recognizing and valuing the efforts parents exert. (Sometimes just acknowledgment that they are working hard on hard issues is enough.)
3. Practicing diplomacy, preferably by learning to be diplomatic in relation to less thorny problems.
4. Listening patiently and well, and using the listening process to pinpoint the root of the problem.
5. Managing any personal sense of hurt, anger, or injustice. (You must be a model of resilience.)
6. Being knowledgeable about parenting resources, as well as ready and willing to refer.
7. Taking risks and trying to anticipate and rise to challenges.

Addressing the accompanying problems in communication counseling is challenging but can be as fulfilling as anything else we do. Box 4–8 provides clinical dilemmas that may lead to interactions with accompanying problems.

## Communication Counselors as Advocates

Jacob is a child with autism. His father has written extensively about Jacob's management for the website, http://www.zerotothree .org. To professionals who might work with Jacob and his family, Jacob's dad gave the following advice:

> Help parents, be sensitive to our needs, but remember who the client is. Don't let us off the hook. Push us, challenge us,

---

### Box 4–8. Exercise: Clinical Dilemmas

Ashton is an autistic 5-year-old. Today, when you were seeing him for language therapy, he bit you on the arm (not hard enough to break the skin through your long-sleeved sweater, but enough to leave a bruise). Ashton's mother was observing the session through a one-way mirror and saw the incident.

- What do you do with Ashton?
- What do you say to his mother?

In another version of this scenario, Ashton's mother was not observing at the time and thus missed the incident. You knew she was not there.

- Does this change what you do with Ashton, or his mother?
- If yes, state the alternatives.

Camille is a 4-year-old child with moderate cerebral palsy. Her mother accompanies her to the therapy room, and when she leaves, Camille begins to cry. You attempt to distract her, but after 10 min, you make no discernible progress.

- What do you do next?
- What do you say to Camille's mother?

At another session, you manage successfully to distract Camille, and she stops crying after a few minutes. At the end of the session, Camille's mother says to you, "How did you do that? It never seems to work for me at home!"

- What do you do or say?

---

keep us on task. We must be a main protagonist if our child is going to get better.

In many communities, the structures and services have not caught up with current innovations and new approaches to intervention. Empower us to be advocates on behalf of our children and embolden us to be subversive when we need to be.

Knowledge and understanding will empower us. Confusion and lack of clarity are disabling. Take the time to explain the issues to us with words we will understand.

Finally, incremental changes in practice and perceptions will not suffice. Rather, a radical paradigm shift concerning the fundamental assumptions regarding who these children with severe disorders in relating and communicating are and what they can accomplish is called for. (From "Jacob's Father," 1997, April/May)

As eloquently stated by Jacob's father, a basic responsibility of communication counselors is to help parents in their quest for the help they perceive they need, and to help them become advocates for their children. As discussed previously, communication counselors are obligated to know the resources available in the community. Particularly important, of course, are parent groups and the opportunities they present for encouraging parents to learn not only from professionals but also from each other. It is also helpful for clinicians to be aware of potential funding sources and pro bono services and opportunities. For example, many communities have strong homeschooling networks. Because of the supports families of homeschoolers need, they have often identified or created local resources that are frequently overlooked and are experienced in advocating to get the supports they value (Duvall, Ward, Delquadri, & Greenwood, 1997; Isenberg, 2007).

## The Internet

As noted in Chapter 2 and throughout examples in this chapter, the Internet is increasingly important for parents as they seek information pertinent to managing their child's disability. Especially useful and reliable sources of such information are the various websites provided by the National Institute of Mental Health (NIMH) and National Institutes of Health (NIH), particularly the websites of the National Institute of Child Health and Development (NICHD) and the National Institute of Deafness and Other Communication Disorders (NIDCD), and those of advocacy organizations such as United Cerebral Palsy, The Arc of the United States, and Family Village, an international resource for persons with disabilities. A number of advocacy sites exist for specific diagnosis and yet the information they have can also be useful for other communication disorders. (See Box 4–9 for examples, and also see the list of Internet resources at the end of this chapter.)

---

**Box 4–9. Maximizing Internet Resources**

Ryan has used information on the construction of Individualized Education Plans published by http://www.autismspeaks.org with parents of children with language impairment. Parents of children with phonological impairments have similarly benefited from information first identified on http://www.chadd.org, a site for children and adults with attention deficit hyperactive disorder. Parents of adolescents who stutter have found their lives as well as their child's life enriched from resources at http://www.authentichappiness.com.

There are many online resources we can carefully vet without becoming so focused on specific disability labels that we fail to see the potential individualized value they may hold for other families. We have found it helpful to keep a counseling folder on our search engines with links to these types of groups. Similarly, communication counselors must be able to assist parents in wading through Internet information to find legitimate advocacy sites.

---

## Networks and Support Groups

Equally important are the growing networks of parent support groups, and the information that parents provide for one another through these networks. A look at self-help websites makes it abundantly clear that many parents have earned their designations as experts in the disorders that affect their children. A sampling of parent support and advocacy websites is provided at the end of the chapter. The listing is not exhaustive in terms of either the problems covered or the extent of good coverage for frequently occurring conditions. An important consideration is that websites must be constantly checked for updates, changes, accuracies, and even disappearances. The listing for this chapter merely includes those websites that currently are among the most parent friendly and provide honest, uplifting information. These websites are easy for parents to access and to participate in their chat rooms and blog sites. These resources allow for benefits of connection with others living with similar challenges. Additionally, communication counselors who find themselves working with clients with specific disorders for which there exist local support groups would do well to establish professional relationships with those running these organizations. It is much easier to advocate for clients and encourage them to participate in support groups when we can personally vouch for the people running the groups.

## A Model of Advocacy

Sue Swenson is a former Director of the Arc of the United States, which is devoted to advocacy and support for persons who have cognitive and intellectual disorders and for their families. She is now at the U.S. Department of Education. The following account of her own experience as the mother of a child with a disability (reproduced from an Arc newsletter, in slightly abridged form) gives her vision of advocacy, which should prove instructive for any counselor who works with parents of children with disabilities.

> When my son Charlie was a baby, the doctor said he was "developmentally delayed." This was a comfort to me, oddly, after months of asking, "What is wrong?" and being told, "There is nothing wrong. Don't compare him to his brother." I didn't know what "developmental delay" meant, but it seemed to mean that I was right to ask if something was wrong. That was a comfort.
>
> The doctor sent me to a brilliant therapist, who told me the truth—that my son's delays were very "significant," that no one could know how everything would turn out, that there were many ways to help him play and have fun with other kids so that his development would not be so affected by his obvious problems. I thought that by talking about hope for his development, she was telling me Charlie's "delays" might go away. I could not imagine and did not have the experience to image that there could be hope with disabilities.
>
> When Charlie was seven, . . . it hit me like a thunderbolt: Charlie's "delays" were not going to go away, and instead of therapy aimed at "fixing" him, he needed inclusive education to make sure that he could make the most out of learning opportunities. He would not be "ready" for school as his class-

mates are ready. But he needed to stop trying to learn stuff that was difficult or impossible to master, like tying his shoes, so that he could move on and learn the important stuff, like how to get along with other people. You can buy shoes with Velcro closures, but there is no Velcro to help you form human attachments.

. . . It is so hard to find the right words to use when talking to parents about disability in children. The future holds so much potential, so much uncertainty, and so much fear. Usually, we parents don't know what it is like to be disabled in America. Unlike most other minorities, we don't often share our child's identifying characteristics.

In my experience, glossing disability over and calling it "delay" doesn't help. It makes parents think that in the end, if we work hard enough, everything will be OK because in the end our child will "catch up." When we are focused on catching up, we don't work on justice for people with disabilities because we don't let ourselves think our children will actually be disabled when they grow up.

No matter what we are told, I think most of us know in our hearts that disabilities are real, and persistent. We, and our children, can be hurt by not letting ourselves think about that reality. We need to learn that hoping, praying, suing, or paying for a "cure" takes away precious time from the real goals of teaching our children that we love them as they are, of helping our children learn how to live well with their disability, and of helping our communities rise to the challenge of justice, decent support and equal access.

Too many children keep getting therapy to help them walk while they get no instruction in how to use a wheelchair; too many keep trying to develop the muscles they need to speak while they get no evaluation for a communication device; too many children spend their school day going from therapy to therapy instead of making friends in their classroom. Too often, children live like this because their parents can't or won't or haven't been encouraged to accept the reality of disability.

Parent advocates have two paths before us: (1) We can use all of our power and parental rights to deny the impending reality of disability, to demand enough therapy to make the "delays" go away; or (2) we can use our voice and our rights to demand justice, access and inclusion for all of our sons and daughters, and to demand recognition of their rights as human beings and as citizens with disabilities. For most parents, advocacy will be a mix of these. Mine was—but experience tells me that it is far better to focus on the latter.

In my experience, many young adults with disabilities are still hoping for their parents to make this leap. In my experience, too many feel their parents are somehow disappointed by their disability, and they feel a righteous anger about this.

We can help our kids if we understand that our sons and daughters are people with disabilities not "delays," and that people with disabilities are people first—whole people first. The sooner we have a chance to learn this, the sooner we can clear up any confusion in our relationships with our children, and the sooner we can say to them, honestly and truthfully: "I see you as you are. I love you as you are. I am proud of you as you are. I will do whatever I can to help you be the best you possible, and I will insist on recognition of your rights."

Maybe then our children can love us as we are, too, although we don't know everything they need to learn, and can't fix everything that may trouble them in life." (Swenson, 2004)

## Bureaucracy

In the United States and other countries, special education laws and laws for human and civil rights have come a long way. There are still many advances that need to be made, some quite desperately; however, with these advances have come bureaucratic creations that can vex the most experienced communication counselors, let alone parents newly confronted with a need to access these systems. We have found in our careers that many times, because parents have been forced into developing their advocacy skills, some of them have become very seasoned in managing these issues. We have learned immensely from them; however, we would like to address how communication counselors can potentially demystify intimidating bureaucratic challenges. Currently, under the Individuals with Disabilities in Education Improvement Act (2004) there is more focus than ever on considering children at risk for or with a disability as member of a family unit and in need of supportive services. This focus recognizes the child's strengths.

Early intervention programs use team models intended to create positive relationships between the family, child, and service providers. Communication counselors working with clients and families receiving early intervention can play a vital role in ensuring that individualized family service plans reflect the values and needs of parents. In these early years, diagnosis and the creation of intervention plans may seem to be a whirlwind of office visits, testing, and paperwork (and the need to quickly acquire a new world of acronyms). Although team models are designed to make sure the family understands and has an appropriate voice in getting their needs met, SLP-As functioning as communication counselors are often in a unique position to sense, and, if necessary, clarify and address, parent concerns. We can help ensure that those involved understand the family's stories and that the signature strengths of parents are acknowledged and, where possible, developed.

Parents of school-aged children are confronted with new models of education and the corresponding bureaucratic vernacular. Currently, a multitier problem-solving approach is in place for ensuring that children receive high-quality instruction and are not inappropriately referred for, or placed in, special education. In public education, it is called response to intervention (RtI) (Damico & Nelson, 2012; Hamayan et al., 2013; Howard, 2009). RtI is intended to provide early flexibility and high-quality culturally and linguistically responsive instruction before special education services are introduced (Allington, 2009). While individual states and school districts typically employ a three-tier model, others accomplish the same general application of the law through models that manifest in four or five tiers (Barnes & Harlacher, 2008). As SLP-As continue to define and implement roles related to these models, our position as communication counselors oriented to wellness and strengths is ideally suited. We can ensure that deficit-based approaches to assessment, which ignore the potential impact of external variables, instructional mismatches, or cultural and linguistic differences, be replaced by more authentic and functional measures (Hamayan, et al., 2013; Howard, 2009). The goal of RtI is to ensure quality of instruction and rule out all other sources of difficulty before the label of disability is applied. Communication counselors can facilitate parents' understanding of RtI while advocating for their child to receive responsive instruction.

Once disability is identified, wellness and strengths-oriented SLP-As can have an impact by advocating for families and ensuring their voices are heard as individualized education programs

(IEPs) are constructed. Through careful preparation and presentation before and during the IEP planning meeting, along with clear documentation of plans and responsibilities, IEPs should become empowering child and family advocating resources.

Unfortunately, parents often do not feel they are full partners in this process (Weishaar, 2010). Only a third of the parents in one study reported being involved in the decision-making process of IEP meetings (Newman, 2005). Parents of older children report even lower levels of involvement and participation (Spann, Kohler, & Soenksen, 2003). Spann, Kohler, and Soenksen (2003) speculate that over time, parents experiencing more conflicts with schools may grudgingly accept what the school imposes on them (Spann et al., 2003; Weishaar, 2010). Friend and Cook (2010) suggest that parental dissatisfaction and lack of involvement in the IEP meeting may stem from feelings of inadequacy of educational knowledge or fear that the questioning of educators may lead to adverse treatment of their children. Communication counselors should be central in addressing these issues. Among the ways in which Weishaar (2010) proposes to better involve parents is to focus on strengths. Box 4–10 presents some examples of how this can be accomplished.

We are not suggesting that we ignore troubles or be dishonest about a child's performance; however, most negative behaviors can be viewed in some positive light. For example, the biting behavior described in Box 4–10 must certainly be addressed and cannot be allowed; however, Jamie has the means of protesting. Even though it is problematic, there is a communicative intent that could be recognized and possibly utilized to develop more appropriate ways of protesting. Strictly lumping her behavior into the bin of "troublemaker" negatively colors Jamie's potential and can dampen the constructive tone needed to develop productive solutions. By beginning IEP meetings with a focus on strengths and ensuring that the child is valued, we can help set the tone of a more positive meeting that is respectful of the child and the parents who want so desperately to help him or her.

Communication counselors can also make sure that parents are aware of the purpose of meetings and what will be discussed. Areas of conflict should be communicated before the meeting so that parents are not blindsided. When they are surprised or shocked with information they are more likely to be forced into a reactionary

---

**Box 4–10. Advocating and Counseling on the IEP Team**

In Chapter 3 we described ways of constructively and destructively responding to concerns. As communication counselors participating in IEP meetings we can set the constructive tone here as well. For example, rather than engaging in destructive responding, we can reframe the presentation by focusing on a child's strengths.

1. Communication counselors can ask IEP team members (including the parents) to prepare a list of the child's strengths and review that list prior to the meeting. So for example:

   ■ Instead of saying, "He can't read on grade level," we might note, "He attentively follows along when he hears others read aloud."

   ■ Rather than dismissing the child as "too lazy to try" or "a cheater," the same behaviors of the child might be recognized as "motivated to be successful." (Although not excusing or advocating cheating, we should consider why a child would expose themselves to the risks and consequences of cheating if they did not care in some way about being successful.)

2. Communication counselors can try to keep discussion oriented to the specific behaviors, even when faced with challenging behaviors such as violence toward other students,

   ■ "Jamie bit her when Christine took her book," rather than broad, sweeping generalizations of value judgments, such as "Jamie is a troublemaker."

---

role and less likely to feel like a collaborator and problem solver. This practice of sharing concerns prior to the meeting should work both ways. As a parent of a child with an IEP, Ryan has been both caught off guard and has caused school personnel to be anxious because of their failure to present concerns before the IEP meeting. In these instances, achieving a collaborative consensus was hampered because of initial defensive reactions. A practice that is too common (and not keeping with the collaborative intent of the meeting) is for SLP-As and other service providers to come to the IEP meeting with their portion of the document already completed with goals and objectives selected from predetermined criteria. While this practice may speed the meeting along, it conveys to parents that their role as a valued team member in the process is diminished. Weishaar (2010) states that clearly labeling the initial IEP paperwork with the word "DRAFT" can also go a long way toward conveying the reality that the meeting is collaborative and the parents' input is needed and important for the final version of the plan. Additionally, we can encourage parents to bring an advocate or other interested party with them to the meeting if they fear they may be overwhelmed. Such encouragement can also signal the importance of ensuring that the parents' voice is heard and their concerns are valued.

In Chapter 3 we described ways of respectfully addressing parents. We would echo that position during IEP meetings. Referring to the child as "kiddo" or to the parents as "mom" or "dad" is not respectful or professional and does not value their strengths and identity. Communication counselors can prepare nametags for people if the meeting is large or participants are not familiar with each other. As current performance is discussed and goals are constructed, the wellness-minded SLP-A should incorporate what the child can *do* when reviewing levels of functioning and considering future objectives. Too often, special education meetings are only about repairing problems. This can be the proverbial salt in an open wound for parents. Communication counselors work to create an environment where trust and respect is fostered so that the parents can feel confident that their child is valued for who they are, and may become, rather than what they have not accomplished.

## Poverty

We feel a strong need to address the issue of poverty and the direct impact it has on counseling and interactions with clients and their families. Our view is that poverty is not merely lack of money; rather, we consider poverty primarily as a lack of opportunities and resources. For example, Ryan has worked with a child who had a very impoverished language-literacy background, yet he came from a family with seemingly unlimited financial resources. He was rarely around other children, and he missed school because his parents traveled so much. They rarely interacted with him during the day and almost never read to or with him; however, once the parents sheepishly recognized what the impact their inattention was having, their substantial resources were enlisted to remediate the situation. On the other hand, we know children from homes with very limited income who, thanks to selfless, resourcefully ingenious parents, never realized the full impact of hard times. We see these two examples as extreme outliers.

Most children who live in poverty experience devastating consequences unfamiliar to most SLP-As. Overwhelmingly, current SLP-As come from white, monolingual, middle-class backgrounds. The link between precipitating conditions and poverty underscores the fact that most clinicians, regardless of ethnic and cultural backgrounds, see many families and children who do not necessarily share their predominantly middle class values and upbringing. This difference in backgrounds has at least as many important ramifications for counseling as for direct intervention. Poverty issues require distinct sensitivity to differing realities of living that are likely to have a direct impact on counseling and interacting with families.

Economic and social class variables are not as well highlighted in our profession's diversity training as ethnic and cultural variables. One result is that economic issues are more invidious than other cross-cultural boundaries for which our training is more explicit. Is Mrs. H late for a session because of a different time perception within her culture, or because of the rigidity of a work schedule that is unsympathetic to the special problems of getting help for an at-risk child? Do one or both parents work at two jobs to make ends meet? If so, does child-rearing become a mutual responsibility for a grandparent as a result? Are there special issues with secondary caregivers? Are our referrals within the realm of financial possibility for a given family? If not, how can we as counselors help families to get needed financial help?

## Communication Counseling with Parents: PERMA Considerations

In Chapter 2 we reviewed the tenets of positive psychology and signature strengths as identified through VIA assessment. As we close this chapter we review the application of what has been presented here from that perspective. Application of PERMA in counseling parents of children at risk for or with communication disorders can and should take many forms. As communication counselors work with parents to help prevent, diagnose, and remediate communication disorders, we can weave these principles into our interactions.

## P: Positive Affect

From a strengths-based perspective, one of our most valuable services may be to help parents see what is right and positive in their lives and learn how to appreciate the value of changes that occur. Educational and medical systems are largely designed to identify deficits and to describe individuals based on comparison with the performance of others. Masked in these rankings are the personal changes that often characterize our clients. In her book *Who's in Charge?*, Susan Ohanian (1994) laments the educational system that fails to recognize the learning that has taken place in a student with language learning impairment and hearing loss. This is because annual yearly progress was not met on the child's standardized test score; however, Ohanian writes, "Leslie read a knock-knock joke to the class with the emphasis in the right place. Anybody who thinks this was a small achievement should've seen the tears of joy streaming down her face and mine as she exclaimed, 'I get it! I really get it! Let me read another one!' . . . or heard her classmates cheering." (Ohanian, 1994, p. 216).

These types of small but very significant positive changes can be highlighted for parents, especially in environments where these qualitative changes might be overlooked. Furthermore, communication counselors can acknowledge and help parents recognize things that they are doing well and the progress they have made.

## E: Engagement (Absorption, Immersion, Flow)

In the context of counseling parents, can we help them understand the importance of finding moments of engagement for themselves as well as that of their children? We have mentioned that parents who are able to experience the rejuvenating power of flow are better able to meet the needs of their children. Additionally, if we assist parents in experiencing and understanding the potential benefits of engagement and flow for their child, perhaps they will better recognize instances when their child is productively absorbed or immersed. In the next chapter, we describe in greater detail what this might look like for children with communication disorders.

## R: Relationships (Involvement with Others, Sharing, Kindness, Being There)

We have described the communication counselor's responsibility for knowing what community resources are available. Furthermore, one of the major benefits of parent support groups is the opportunity they afford for the development of relationships. SLP-As can help parents recognize and accentuate VIA signature strengths in the relationships that they have. As we come to know a parent's story we should be able to help them identify relationships where they might grow their strengths and virtues. We can then better mediate these attributes when parents experience potential misinterpretations of messages. Communication counselors functioning as models of how to reframe negative interactions, and individuals willing to take time to allow parents opportunities to share, can facilitate flourishing relationships.

## M: Meaning (Belonging to or Serving Something Bigger Than Oneself)

As we work with parents, we might review the themes of meaning that were presented in Chapter 2. Communication counselors can assist parents in reflecting on what brought meaning to their life prior to their child's manifestation of the communication disorder. Is there any way similar elements could be brought forward again? For example, are there support networks or respite services that can be accessed to allow parents opportunities for moments to revisit or reengage in those meaningful activities in some way? Are there new groups or activities that would allow parents to build upon their strengths? What new opportunities are available for them to develop commitments that can transform their lives? Which of their signature strengths could be used to develop new commitments. For parents who struggle to see the forest of possibility through the overwhelming trees of struggle, again, communication counselors might help parents address the following three questions: (1) What commitments to a meaningful life were in place before the catastrophe? (2) How can they be optimized? and (3) Can new commitments emerge as the result of this potentially transformative experience? Support groups and advocacy organizations are often helpful in these situations. Most groups never have enough volunteers for the service they try to render. These are ready-made opportunities for parents of children with a disability to connect and contribute to something larger.

### A: Accomplishment (Pursuing and Achieving a Goal for Its Own Sake)

The strategies we have discussed for discovering a parent's story from their perspective is vital for SLP-As to provide counsel in this area. As parents cope and adjust to the consequences and impact of the labels placed on their children, their hopes and dreams may be dramatically realigned. A communication counselor's ability to help parents identify signature strengths and work to grow them can do much to aid in this redirecting or recalibration. These reconstructed goals and aspirations can be better defined and plans to achieve them can be more clearly established. Communication counselors can help parents realize how day-to-day goals are contributing to the greater accomplishments that parents envision.

## Conclusion

We have articulated in this chapter many of the concerns and considerations that parents of children at risk for communication disorders may experience. We have tried to provide strategies for how SLP-As can adopt a wellness perspective in the communication counseling of parents in these situations. Our examples are not perfect but hopefully they are enough to get you thinking about your own counseling moments with parents and how you can use their signature strengths to flourish. It might be valuable to reflect on a specific parent from your clinical practice. What might you guess are their signature strengths (see again the list in Chapter 2)? What is another way you could have helped them use that specific strength in a recent counseling moment? In the next chapter we shift from a focus on parent interaction to considerations for providing communication counseling to children with communication disorders.

# References

Allington, R. L. (2009). *What really matters in response to intervention: Research-based designs.* Boston, MA: Allyn & Bacon.

Balint, M. (1957). *The doctor, his patient, and the illness.* New York, NY: International Universities Press.

Barnes, A. C., & Harlacher, J. E. (2008). Clearing the confusion: Response-to-intervention as a set of principles. *Education and Treatment of Children, 31,* 417–431.

Caesar, L. G., & Kohler, P. D. (2007). The state of school-based bilingual assessment: Actual practice versus recommended guidelines. *Language, Speech, and Hearing Services in Schools, 38*(3), 190–200.

Connor, D. (2006). Michael's story: "I get into so much trouble just by walking": Narrative knowing and life at the intersections of learning disability, race, and class. *Equity & Excellence in Education, 39*(2), 154–165.

Connor, D. J., & Ferri, B. A. (2005). Integration and inclusion: A troubling nexus. Race, disability, and special education. *Journal of African American History, 90*(1/2), 107–127.

Damico, J. S., & Augustine, L. E. (1995). Social considerations in the labeling of students as attention deficit hyperactivity disordered. *Seminars in Speech and Language, 16,* 259–274.

Damico, J. S., Muller, N., & Ball, M. J. (2010). Social and practical considerations in labeling. In J. S. Damico, N. Muller, & M. J. Ball (Eds.), *The handbook of language and speech disorders.* Oxford, UK: Blackwell.

Damico, J. S., & Nelson, R. L. (2012). Response to intervention. In E. Hamayan & R. Freeman (Eds.), *English language learners at school. A guide for administrators.* Philadelphia, PA: Caslon.

Damico, J. S., & Simmons-Mackie, N. N. (2003). Qualitative research and speech-language pathology: Impact and promise in the clinical realm. *American Journal of Speech Language Pathology, 12,* 131–143.

Dudley-Marling, C. (2000). *A family affair: When school troubles come home.* Portsmouth, NH: Heinemann.

Duvall, S. F., Ward, D. L., Delquadri, J. C., & Greenwood, C. R. (1997). An exploratory study of home school instructional environments and their effects on the basic skills of students with learning disabilities. *Education and Treatment of Children, 20*, 150–172.

Fraiberg, S., Adelson, E., & Shapiro, V. (1975). Ghosts in the nursery: A psychoanalytic approach to the problem of impaired infant-mother relationships. *Journal of the American Academy of Child Psychiatry, 14*, 799–803.

Friend, M., & Cook, L. (2010). *Interactions: Collaboration skills for school professionals* (6th ed.). Upper Saddle River, NJ: Pearson.

Gergen, K. J. (2001). *Social construction in context*. London, UK: Sage.

Gergen, K. J. (2008). *An invitation to social construction*. London, UK: Sage.

Gergen, K. J. (2009). *Relational being: Beyond self and community*. New York, NY: Oxford University Press.

Gillman, M., Heyman, B., & Swain, J. (2000). What's in a name? The implications of diagnosis for people with learning difficulties and their family carers. *Disability and Society, 15*(3), 389–409.

Goffman, E. (1964). *Stigma: Notes on the management of spoiled identity*. New York, NY: Simon and Schuster.

Greenspan, S. I. (2001). *The secure child: Helping our children feel safe and confident in a changing world*. Cambridge, MA: First Da Capo Press.

Grinker, R. (2007). *Unstrange minds: Remapping the world of autism*. Cambridge, MA: Basic Books.

Hamayan, E., Marler, B., Sanchez-Lopez, C., & Damico, J. (2013). *Special education considerations for English language learners*. Philadelphia, PA: Caslon.

Heinrichs, R. (2003). *Perfect targets: Apserger syndrome and bullying*. Shawnee Mission, KS: Autism Asperger Publishing.

Heise, D. R. (2007). *Expressive order: Confirming sentiments in social actions*. New York, NY: Springer.

Howard, M. (2009). *RTI from all sides: What every teacher needs to know*. Portsmouth, NH: Heinemann.

Individuals with Disabilities in Education Improvement Act, PL 108-4 66. (2004). 20 USC 1400.

Isenberg, E. J. (2007). What have we learned about homeschooling? *Peabody Journal of Education, 82*, 387–409.

"Jacob's Father." (1997, April/May). *Jacob's story: A miracle of the heart*. Retrieved from http://www.zerotothree.org

Kelly, N., & Norwich, B. (2004). Pupils' perceptions of self and of labels: Moderate learning difficulties in mainstream and special schools. *British Journal of Educational Psychology, 74*(3), 411–435.

Kroska, A., & Harkness, S. K. (2008). Exploring the role of diagnosis in the modified labeling theory of mental illness. *Social Psychology Quarterly, 71*(2), 193–208.

Laminack, L., & Wadsworth, R. (2012). *Bullying hurts: Teaching kindness through read alouds and guided conversations.* Portsmouth, NH: Heinemann.

Newman, L. (2005). Family expectations and involvement for youth with disabilities. *National Longitudinal Transition Study 2 Data Brief, 4,* 1–5.

Ohanian, S. (1994). *Who's in charge?* Portsmouth, NH: Boynton/Cook/ Heinemann.

Parr, S., Byng, S., Gilpin, S., & Ireland, C. (1997). *Talking about aphasia: Living with loss of language following stroke.* Buckingham, UK: Open University Press.

Sharry, J. (2004). *Counselling children, adolescents, and families.* London, UK: Sage.

Simmons-Mackie, N. N., & Damico, J. S. (2003). Contributions of qualitative research to the knowledge base of normal communication. *American Journal of Speech-Language Pathology, 12,* 144–154.

Smith, F. (1998). *The book of learning and forgetting.* New York, NY: Teachers College Press.

Solomon, A. (2012). *Far from the tree.* New York, NY: Scribner.

Spann, S. J., Kohler, F. W., & Soenksen, D. (2003). Examining parents' involvement in and perceptions of special education services: An interview with families in a parent support group. *Focus on Autism and Other Developmental Disabilities, 18,* 228–237.

Spradley, J. P. (1979). *The ethnographic interview.* New York, NY: Holt, Rhinehart & Winston.

Stillman, R., Snow, R., & Warren, K. (1999). "I used to be good with kids." Encounters between speech-language pathology students and children with PDD. In D. Kovarsky, J. Duchan, & M. Maxwell (Eds.), *The social construction of language incompetence.* Hillside, NJ: Lawrence Erlbaum Associates.

Swenson, S. (2004). Newsletter of the Arc of the United States.

Trelease, J. (2006). *The read-aloud handbook* (6th ed.). New York, NY: Penguin Books.

Weishaar, P. M. (2010). What's new in . . . Twelve ways to incorporate strengths-based planning into the IEP process. *Clearing House, 83,* 207–210.

Westby, C. E. (1990) Ethnographic interviewing: Asking the right questions to the right people in the right ways. *Journal of Childhood Communication Disorders, 13,* 101–111.

# Websites

The following websites were chosen primarily because they are those of advocacy groups or otherwise addressed to parents, and because they provide links to other websites of interest. Only a few sites per disorder are provided, although there are many more. Using a search engine, such as Google, and entering the relevant search term for each disorder listed here, as well as many others, will yield specific technical information. Generally, such information is clearly available under the refined search term "health professionals." Communication counselors should be particularly careful to check websites periodically for their relevance, factual content, and currency. Also, it is important to pay frequent visits to the various NIH/NIMH[2] websites for updates.

## Specific Disorder Focus

Autism spectrum disorders:

> http://www.kylestreehouse.org
>
> http://www.maapservices.org
>
> http://www.autismspeaks.org

Cerebral palsy:

> http://www.originsofcerebralpalsy.com
>
> http://www.ucp.org

Cleft palate and other craniofacial anomalies:

> http://www.widesmiles.org
>
> http://www.apert.org
>
> http://www.faces-cranio.org
>
> http://www.friendlyfaces.org

---

[2]National Institutes of Health/National Institute of Mental Health.

Down syndrome:

    http://www.ndss.org

    http://www.bandofangels.com

Learning disabilities:

    http://www.ldonline.org

    http://www.ricklavoie.com

Hearing:

    http://www.handsandvoices.org

    http://www.beginningssvcs.com

## General

    http://www.familyvillage.wisconsin.edu

    http://www.thearc.org

    http://www.zerotothree.org

    http://www.loc.gov/bookfest/kids-teachers

    http://www.trelease-on-reading.com

    http://www.bigpicture.org

    http://www.edutopia.org

## English Language Learners

    http://www.wida.us

## Information from Books Oriented to Children

    http://www.mowillems.com

    http://www.pilkey.com

http://www.juniebjones.com

http://www.magictreehous.com

# Chapter 5

# COUNSELING ISSUES WITH CHILDREN WHO HAVE COMMUNICATION DISORDERS

"*Dakota*" was a 16-year-old high school student when she wrote the following account of her early life experiences as a young person who stutters:

> After my sixth grade year, I decided that I couldn't let my stuttering stop me anymore. I was going to junior high school in a few months and it was time to start being like all the other kids. Then, two years ago I joined the marching band at my high school. We went to band camp, and I met a lot of new people, and nobody paid attention to my stuttering. This was the first time in my life that people didn't treat me different because of my stuttering. That was also when I realized that my stuttering really didn't matter to other people. In fact, my band teacher had been my teacher for two years and didn't even know I stuttered until just this past year.

Now that I'm in high school, I really don't enjoy getting up in front of people and giving speeches, but everyone has to do some things in life they don't want to do. I love to talk. I spend most of my time out of school on the phone, and I've made a whole lot of friends. I'm now very outspoken. I don't hide any of my emotions anymore. I tell people what's on my mind, and when I want to talk, I do. When I'm having a bad day, I stutter more than I do when I have a good day. But sometimes days go by when I don't stutter at all, and it makes me feel great.

I hope this letter inspires many people my age. I hope younger children can learn that they are not the only ones out there who stutter, and that they can stand up for themselves. I had a fantastic speech teacher when I was in elementary school. She was willing to listen to what I had to say, and she taught me how to deal with my stuttering. She was a great person.

Don't worry if people make fun of you. They can't help it. I used to get angry when people would laugh at me, but that's one thing you just have to ignore in life. Don't let anyone tell you that you can't do something because you stutter; you can do whatever you feel like doing and saying. My stuttering used to have a great impact on my life, but now I have learned to work around it. (*Source:* The National Stuttering Association)

## Introduction

Counseling opportunities frequently arise in our interactions with children who have communication disorders; however, they may take different forms and require different approaches from those we described in Chapter 4. Variables such as developmental level, degree of cognitive and linguistic functioning, and the type and severity of impairment all come into play as counseling moments occur. In addition, those factors also affect the manner in which SLP-A's go about their counseling. Some of our work with preschoolers and children in elementary schools may not seem to be counseling at times. Nevertheless, our work should help children to feel valued as we help them to develop strategies for overcoming, compensate for, and adapt to challenges, build resilience and capitalize on strengths in order to grow and live as fully as possible.

The focus of this chapter is on how the "quiet" and "loud" counseling characteristics (see Chapter 3) and interactional strategies of SLP-As can meet these goals.

## Reframing Behavior: Finding Strength

In the previous chapter we discussed some ways to reframe issues in SLP-A meetings and interactions with parents. Reframing is also important in direct work with children who have communication disorders. Important as it is to be able to diagnose and manage speech, language, and hearing problems, orientation to wellness in counseling children requires us to identify their strengths and help them to move forward. It requires us to recognize the affect that underlies and motivates current behaviors, and we must have a willingness to embrace the child as a respected and valued inter-active partner, even in the face of limited communication skills.

Box 5–1 summarizes a counseling issue from clinical interactions with an adolescent with diagnosed communication disorders. As an exercise, read the summary and reflect on the bulleted points.

It is easy to imagine some of the struggles that clinicians working with Jose encountered as they tried to help him meet therapy goals and objectives in succeeding sessions. We can envision the difficulties the next clinician working with him might have encountered in trying to convince Jose that he could make progress and that he was valued as a communicator. The efforts of his next clinician to help Jose identify and build upon strengths were certainly not enhanced by his experience in witnessing how those who should care the most viewed him. Ultimately, we can imagine that counseling moments would most certainly appear in his future speech-language therapy sessions; however, some subtle but powerful and potentially supportive strengths are reflected in Jose's behavior.

While the adults talked about Jose, he did his best to become invisible and disappear. A wellness- or strengths-oriented communication counselor might interpret the act of pulling his jacket over his head and trying to turn away as indicating that Jose understood that the situation was not positive. Furthermore, one could infer from his attempts to disappear that he truly cared about what others thought of him and, clearly, that he would rather be viewed favorably.

## Box 5–1. Recognizing and Reframing

Read the following story and reflect on the questions that follow:

"Jose" was a 12-year-old sixth grade student in a self-contained classroom in a rural public school in the south. His parents were involved in a messy divorce with Jose and his two much younger siblings caught in the middle. He had been diagnosed early in his education with a variety of labels from both the medical and educational communities. Jose's labels included moderate learning disability, moderate-severe language disorder, attention deficit hyperactivity disorder, and dyslexia. One February, after lunch, he was called from his classroom to participate in his Individualized Education Program meeting. His mother thought he should be present for the meeting and school officials obliged her. They wanted Jose to begin taking greater responsibility for his actions and his education. In some situations, such an idea may be very helpful and empowering for the child. This was not such a situation.

Jose had recently had an outburst on the bus ride to school and the IEP team was gathering to consider modification to his placement and the special education supports he was receiving. The motivating event prompting this reconvening occurred when he threatened to harm a student, Cody, who was wheelchair-bound, nonverbal, and very low functioning. Jose perceived that Cody was making fun of the way he was dressed. Given Cody's diagnosis and level of functioning, the reality was more likely that he was just giggling. Cody often giggled and laughed for no easily observable reason. This time, however, he happened to make eye contact with Jose at the same time. Jose had lashed out verbally, threatening violence (something to the effect of, "Shut-up, Cody, or I'll hit you—I mean it!" The bus driver was shocked and concerned that Jose would be so aggressive toward a much more defenseless child. A conduct referral was made with the recommendation that Jose receive harsh consequences for this unprovoked act of aggression. This event, plus the fact that Jose was continuing to struggle academically, prompted the IEP meeting.

Upon joining the meeting, Jose listened as his mother, teachers, and school administrators described his behavior and educational shortcomings. Examples of his many struggles were detailed. Expulsion from the school and reassignment to an alternative, disciplinary school was being proposed. The school counselor and the SLP both thought that such a move was hasty and both tried to describe the progress Jose was making, as well as to illustrate all that Jose was learning to accomplish. They voiced real concern with the notion of changing Jose's educational placement. Through all this negotiation, the adults in the room failed to recognize that Jose was slowly pulling his jacket up over his head and physically trying to silently turn away from the group. This was a horrible, degrading, and demeaning experience for Jose. Mercifully, the counselor, suddenly aware of the affective signals Jose was communicating, got up and invited him to join her in an activity outside of the room. The SLP also belatedly recognized what was going on and, as soon as Jose and the counselor left the room, she brought it to the attention of the rest of the team. The meeting quickly ended, but not before expulsion and recommendations for greater behavioral modification were made and Jose was left to receive his education and special education services at the alternative, disciplinary school.

We can easily find in this glimpse of a clinical situation a number of problems and lapses in professional and parental judgment. The ethics, legalities, and certainly the humanity underscoring how Jose was treated could and should be called into question. In fact, Jose's father, contending that his son's right to a free and appropriate education in the least restrictive environment had been impinged upon, later brought the matter before the courts. Unfortunately, two years after this IEP meeting, Jose had dropped out of school and services altogether. This story also allows for some reflection on potential communication counseling opportunities with a child.

- What type of counseling moments might arise from this experience with Jose?
- Is Jose aware of his struggles? What behaviors tell you this?
- Can Jose's behaviors be reframed in a more positive light?
- Where would you start as a communication counselor confronted with this situation?

Although not the most productive, conventional, or age-appropriate way to do that, Jose was strategically communicating, at least to his counselor and SLP, that he was having an emotionally painful experience. Jose created the strategies of turning away and pulling his jacket over his head. We should recognize that if Jose can independently create *any* communicative strategies (albeit not very effective ones), he could be supported and encouraged to develop more productive ones.

Damico and Nelson (2005) described compensatory strategies in children with communication disorders as attempts they make to meet the communicative and cognitive demands placed upon them despite their limitations. Perkins (2005) writes that when interactional demands exceed an individual's capacities for successful communication, what emerges are systematic, individually specific compensations that, in some way, fulfill the communicative demands. These interactional strategies are not necessarily consciously created; rather, children are simply doing what they can in the given situation. In children with communication disorders, these adaptations are not always efficient or appropriate for the context, but they do reflect the best that the person can do at that specific moment (Damico & Nelson, 2005; Herrera, Smith, Nelson, & Abendroth, 2009; Perkins, 2001, 2005; Rydell, 2012).

## Reframing Compensatory Strategies

Often, the compensatory strategies that children with communication disorders create appear maladaptive for the interactional or educational setting. On the surface, these strategies look like problematic behaviors that interfere with the child's opportunities for success. Communication counselors should seek to look beyond the maladaptive nature of the behavior and understand the underlying motivation that generates the need for creating a strategy. For example, when a clinician asks a child with a communication disorder and reading difficulties to read aloud to the class, the child may engage in avoidance behaviors such as off-task commenting and actions, excessive talking about topics related to the story, rereading material previously covered, or even overt refusals to read. On the surface, these behaviors may be undesirable. Furthermore, the child's creation and use of such strategies prevents them from benefiting from instruction. However, reframing the behavior from a strengths perspective can reveal how the child is meeting a communicative demand despite their struggles (Damico, Abendroth, Nelson, Lynch, & Damico, 2011). From children's perspective, when they are asked to do something they do not know how to do or do not want to do, their "problematic" responses may seem to them to be a better option than appearing incompetent.[1] Armed with this understanding, communication counselors can monitor interactions and better support the child. For instance, the clinician can ensure that struggling readers not be asked to read aloud to the class material that they have not had a prior opportunity to practice. This would minimize the potential embarrassment for the child and eliminate his or her need for the compensatory strategy that appears to be maladaptive.

In children with communication disorders, compensatory strategies that look to us as disruptive or inappropriate may make assessments and interventions quite challenging (Damico et al., 2011; Damico et al., 2008; Damico & Nelson, 2005; Perkins, 2001, 2005). Communication counselors oriented to wellness recognize that they may represent strengths. For example, the deployment of strategies of any kind may suggest that children who use them are aware of the social role they are expected to fulfill. Compensatory strategies can also indicate that the child has a capacity to *construct* strategies, effective or not. Revisiting Jose's situation, he was never taught that pulling his jacket over his head and turning away was a communicative strategy. As communication counselors, we can consider the possibility that if a Jose or another child can come up with less productive strategies on their own, with our help they should be able to develop more effective, efficient, and appropriate strategies. Reframing can have a powerful impact on a communication counselor's ability to help a child move forward.

## Quiet Technical Skills

### *Maintaining Expectations*

We discussed the impact of labeling on parents in Chapter 4. Labels also have an impact on the children with whom we work. SLP-As

---

[1] Isn't this true of all of us adults as well?

should not define children's potential by diagnostic labels; rather, they must focus on actual proficiency. Because most educational systems are set up as competitive arenas, children's communicative limitations are glaringly apparent and make it taxing but still necessary to maintain positive expectations for growth and development. Most child-oriented SLP-As struggle to find success socially and/ or academically for their children. The challenge for communication counselors is to be able to recognize strengths while balancing realistic expectations in light of the communication disorder. Clinical skill in reframing behaviors from a strengths perspective is a necessary, but not sufficient, skill. We talked earlier about the importance of our professional knowledge base concerning diagnosis and projected changes over time. In addition, clinicians must become skilled in recognizing what a problem looks like in real life. This involves recognizing the impact of contextual variables and social demands and how they may change over time.

Will Kenny, a very early stutterer, be among the 80% of stuttering children who become normal speakers, or will his stuttering continue despite therapy and be an influential factor in his adult life? Will Janet, who has specific language impairment, become a normal language user, or will she remain challenged by language and learning disabilities throughout her life? With traumatic brain injury, what are the long-term consequences, not only for Barry, who has a severe head injury, but also for Barbra, whose head injury was comparatively mild? Will Barry ever be able to manage on his own, or will he always be dependent on others to survive? Will Barbara be able to complete high school or go to college? Will Matthew, who has autism, be able to develop emotional regulation so that transitions are not so challenging. Will he ever develop and experience the joys of friendships with peers? Will Sam ever be able to conventionally communicate his needs? A wellness perspective can serve as a balance to expectations, because it avoids the inherent contradictions between "who the child is" and "what his or her label is."

Even though children may not say so or even explicitly consider it, effective communication counselors attempt to move beyond the "Popeye approach"—that is, "I am what I am, a person with a communicative disorder. I have to learn to live with it, and you must accept me as I am." A wellness perspective is more akin to the following: "For me, I just *am*. I will change what I can and learn to live with what I cannot. I need to move on, beyond an identity of being someone with a communication disorder. I am someone who can grow and develop in uniquely fascinating ways and you should expect nothing less than that from me." This perspective does not ignore the child's challenges; rather, it seeks to embrace his or her potential with an appreciation that their trajectory of development will be unique and wonderful.

It is important to work within the framework of what we can and cannot fix. If we attempt to change the unchangeable, we risk running aground on a sea of failed expectations; however, worrying about the future is the major ingredient of anxiety, and forecasting negative outcomes for disorders is a tricky and difficult business. (You will read more about these issues for adults in Chapters 6 and 7). The progression of most communication disorders of childhood is unique to the child and his or her experiences. The counseling issues that arise can be as challenging as those encountered in counseling parents. For example, after a particularly difficult session, it may be hard to envision the child with a substantial language disorder who is struggling to read in third grade, going on to graduate education; however, this happens (Kasten, 1998). Fink (1995) described individuals diagnosed with severe dyslexia who were viewed by their teachers as unlikely to acquire reading proficiency. This study described how these bleak futures were transformed into substantial successes. The need for optimism and resilience is as great especially when so much of life lies ahead. For children whose problems are skewed toward the severe end of each disorder's continuum, resilience and optimism may be difficult to achieve; however, communication counselors should still be able to assist these children in feeling valued, secure, and able to experience life to their fullest potential.

Later in the book (Chapter 9), Stan Goldberg describes the role of SLP-As in working with clients who are close to death. Following a lecture, Goldberg was asked how a clinician can feel successful when ultimately their client's health deteriorates to the point of death. He responded that his role in these situations was not to cure or improve; rather, he was there to help them live with dignity and as fully as their situation allowed. There is valuable wisdom in this perspective, which also applies to working with children with communication disorders. As SLP-As adopt a more child-centered approach to learning children's strengths, they provide the child with an opportunity to flourish and to feel and develop a sense of dignity. In Ryan's first year as a full-time public school clinician, his CFY supervisor, Mary Lobdell, constantly reminded him, "From most parents' perspective and certainly most children's perspective, if they leave a clinical interaction believing, 'Mr. Ryan sure knows I'm worth something,' then you have probably earned your keep." Children who feel valued and experience positive relationships are more willing to engage in the hard work of improving their communication patterns (Greenspan, 2001; Seligman, 2011).

## *Waiting*

The ability to observe and recognize the patterns of preference, favored activities, tendencies, quirks, and relevant personality traits in the children we work with does much to facilitate our capabilities as counselors (Fox, 2008). This requires expertise in applying both the quiet and loud technical skills described in Chapter 3, specifically in our interactions with children. We now focus on the application of the quieter skills.

At the beginning of this chapter, Dakota described the qualities of her speech teacher. It is probably not a coincidence that the first attribute she listed was the clinician's willingness to listen. It was not the scientifically defensible technique (though that was surely important as well); rather, it was the quiet skill of a clinician's ability to listen that resonated with this child years later.

Many children SLP-As work with have communication disorders that show themselves in behaviors that have a significant impact on the efficiency of both processing and communicating information. It is easy to see this in some children, for example, those with autism. With autistic children, a common intervention strategy is to use minimal speech and proximal communication (Potter & Whittaker, 2001). Clinicians use this technique by minimizing their own speech with the intent to avoid overwhelming the child's regulatory system and allow them to complete the task (Prelock, 2006). Potter and Whittaker (2001) suggest that clinicians should use clearly contrastive bursts of talking with moments of relatively passive communication, allowing the child an opportunity to process and respond. To this end, communication counselors understand the importance of silence. The importance of being heard and allowed the opportunity to state one's ideas is key.

Rydell (2012) comments that too often SLP-As act during therapy as though they are being paid by the words they say.[2] Our wish to assist and minimize potential frustration can lead us to prompt, reissue directions, or change the task before the child has either processed or been able to formulate a response. Overeagerness to step in[3] may prevent children from using self-monitoring strategies or corrective strategies that will be necessary when they confront similar situations when the clinician is not present. As noted earlier, pausing is a difficult thing to learn, for lots of reasons starting with our own tendencies to fill silences with words, but with children, we may also worry that they are avoiding the task or may simply be confused. To be sure, knowing just how long to wait is an art; however, orienting to wellness, assuming that children are predisposed to social appropriateness, and adopting something akin to counting to at least five can function as a powerful intervention strategy. Communication counselors must remember that what may seem like a long time for an adult may not be enough for a child (Oldfather, Bonds, & Bray, 1994). When we add a communication impairment that includes some cognition problems or difficulty in the efficiency of communication, the need for more time to respond increases.

### Listening to the Stories

Considering the quieter skills communication counselors must develop, it is prudent to revisit listening to stories from the perspective of the child. Stories are as clinically relevant for them as they are for their parents. As children learn to build narratives, they learn to make sense of their experiences and acquire much of their linguistic and communicative proficiency (Ochs, 2004). Older children and adolescents also have their own stories to tell. The basic reasons for encouraging stories remain the same for both children and adults, but there are additional considerations for children. As children convey their stories they are also engaging in developmental work that expands cognitive structures (Wells, 1999, 2001),

---

[2]Adult clinicians have this tendency, too. Audrey's spouse once asked for, and was given, permission to watch one of my sessions with an adult who stuttered. After it was over, he asked (not unkindly) how I expected him to improve when I did all the talking! OOPS!

[3]The 5-second rule applies to everybody, too!

simultaneously expressing their perspective on their experiences. The communication counselor who encourages stories should not limit them to only the "bad stuff" (McCabe & Peterson, 1984; McCabe & Rollins, 1994). To maximize the positive and explore and shape resilience and optimism, stories about what is going well are at least as important as the painful ones. That being said, because of the trust that is often formed between SLP-As oriented toward valuing a child's stories, communication counselors must be ready and willing to listen carefully and responsively when children reveal the "bad stuff."

When creating opportunities for children to share their stories and while engaged in the process of listening to stories, SLP-As must again resist the urge to correct or quickly address aspects of the story that are not germane to understanding what the child is trying to share. If the purpose is hearing what is being conveyed through the story, then that is where the focus should be. Most clinicians would not monitor and correct grammatical or even semantic errors in nonimpaired adults or children unless those errors created substantial confusion. Yet when a child is on our caseload, a dominant interpretive framework is that form is prioritized over the intended message (Damico & Damico, 1997). We tend not to do this when we encourage stories from parents. If we want to be effective counselors, we must make content the priority with their children as well.

Remember that the stimulus for getting people to tell their stories is simply to ask to hear them. In assessment and in subsequent individual sessions, counselors need to identify the disorienting dilemmas stories may contain and recognize the opportunities they provide for growth and change. In groups, the storytelling process presents opportunities to learn from others as well through the authentic and supportive responses of group members.

The importance of stories is a central theme throughout this book. Another benefit of the quiet skill of eliciting and listening to stories are the positive and unique effects storytelling has on children's cognitive development. Nelson (1989, 2003) argues that reflecting on and sharing personal stories with someone who is genuinely interested helps children create the cognitive structures necessary for learning how to organize and make sense of their future experiences. Communication counselors recognize a vital importance of stories for both cognitive development and for establishing resilience. As children seek to understand their experiences through storytelling, they can try out different problem-solving strategies and build cognitive power necessary for dealing with future challenges (Feldman, 1989). Part of the power of stories comes from others' authentic reactions to what is shared and how it is conveyed. As stories are repeated, even if they are not entirely accurate, the importance that a specific story holds in our lives increases and can ultimately shape how we view who we are (Egan, 1995; Hardcastle, 2003). It also increases the significant impact communication counselors can have on children. As SLP-As learn to elicit and promote stories in clinical situations, the counseling moments that emerge can be better utilized.

The ethnographic interviewing strategies and techniques for inviting stories described in Chapter 4 can be applied here as well. Stories also can be used as a basis for intervention. For example, Paley (1994a, 1994b) encouraged communicatively impaired children from linguistically and culturally diverse backgrounds to tell their stories to each other in a classroom setting. The goal was to facilitate peer acceptance. With the teacher's help as required, all the class members wrote either true or imaginary stories and then shared them with the others. Next, the stories were acted out by other class members, with the author-child retaining proprietary rights including the right to determine whether or not the interpretation was acceptable. When the author-child judged the acting out to be unacceptable, he or she then was able to function as a "natural-born" storyteller. Furthermore, the others were engaged and supportive. Paley's approach capitalizes more on the counselor's listening skills, rather than have the counselor be responsible for generating and constructing the story.

## Loud Technical Skills

### Responses

The louder counseling skills SLP-As frequently employ usually occur following a child's communication attempt. Cambourne (1988) studied children in academic settings and suggested eight key principles contributing to how learning can occur naturally, efficiently, and in a way that is both functionally relevant for them and does not fade over time. Like Cambourne, we use learning to read and write as our example of the following principles:

- *Immersion*—Learners need to be immersed in whatever phenomenon they are attempting to acquire. With reading and writing this principle would be realized by saturating the child's environment with a wide variety of examples (books, magazines, signs, e-mail, note, grocery lists, etc.)

- *Demonstration*—A learner should have a lot of opportunities to see how reading and writing genres are created and used. For example, children need to see how we use reading and writing throughout our day. How do we decide what goes on our grocery list? How do we decide if we want to read a certain book? How are poetry, fiction, and nonfiction used? How does someone make word meaning or grammar choices as he or she writes?

- *Expectation*—The experienced reader and writer must expect that the child will, at some point, learn to do the same. There should be an underlying belief that the potential for learning to read and write exists and that the child is on the path to becoming proficient.

- *Responsibility*—Learners need to be allowed to make many of their own choices about when, how, and what parts of the phenomenon they will learn. The more competent readers and writers believe children will take responsibility for learning as they acquire more experience and develop greater control of strategies and are allowed to use them for authentic reading and writing tasks.

- *Use*—Learners must have a chance to use their reading and writing abilities independently for real purposes. They should be allowed to practice reading books they select, writing stories on topics they select. This practice should be uncontrolled, functional, and realistic, closely resembling the reading and writing uses of proficient readers and writers.

- *Approximations*—As learners participate and practice, mistakes should both be expected and allowed. Unfortunately, approximations are often viewed by clinicians or educators as errors that are to be punished and extinguished, rather than viewing them as a natural process of organizing and testing the learner's mental hypothesis (see the reframing discussion above). A simple example will illustrate the all too common reluctance to appreciate approximations for what they tell us about what the child can do: Suppose a clinician was going to consider a child's spelling ability. The child is asked to spell the word "sat" and she produces "C-A-T" (a possible compensatory strategy). Of course the word is not spelled in the conventional manner; however, the child's approximation is much closer than if they had produced numbers or even something like "TTTT." Operating from an assumption that children typically would rather be successful leads communication counselors to look for an underlying logic or rationale for behavior that reflects strength and capacity (two out of three ain't bad!). It is not hard to understand how "C-A-T" for "sat" may have materialized. It can reveal what strategies the child was using as he or she attempted to meet the request.

■ *Response*—Our reluctance to appreciate the approximation principle is typically observed in how we react to a child's attempts at using the phenomenon being learned. How we respond to the child's attempts as they try to make connections to their background experience and to refine their abilities often directly influences whether or not we can help them. Our feedback must be helpful, functional, timely, and nonthreatening. The feedback, support, or instruction we provide should be offered to help the child make sense of the story in the moment they need it to better tackle whatever they are reading or writing.

■ *Engagement*—Although it is presented last, engagement is necessary with each of the previous principles of learning and is key to the success of a child's development. With reading and writing, communication counselors use their loud technical skills with the response principle. If the responses that children receive for their approximations are negative, they will be less likely to engage and continue to take risks. Kohn (1993) notes that when accuracy in performance is the pervasive focus, children also become alienated and lose interest in acquiring whatever is being taught. Consequently, we will not be able to provide instruction that is relevant at a teachable moment. Furthermore, as

Smith (1998) suggests in *The Book of Learning and Forgetting*, we have learned how to teach children many things but the one thing we have not been able to teach is how to forget. This becomes important if our responses to a child's approximations teaches them that they are not valued members of the group of individuals capable of doing the specific phenomenon.

## Impact of Responses

Cambourne's principles have been successfully applied to responsiveness and engagement with children who have ADHD (Nelson & Hawley, 2004) and are potentially appropriate for children who have other communication disorders. Communication counselors can carefully consider the nature and use of their responses. Beyond keeping children engaged, the responses produced by SLP-As to children, even when positive, can sometimes create unintended consequences. Kohn (2001) describes potential consequences of verbal praise when it is applied too frequently and haphazardly. Reflecting on the negative consequences of doling out the phrase "Good job!" in response to a child's behavior can lead to at least five not necessarily intended consequences. First, consider who benefits from verbal praise. When a client cleans up the Play-Doh after a session and is treated with "Good job cleaning up!" it is possible that this has more to do with our convenience than with meeting the needs of the child. In this way Kohn suggests that praise can be a form of *manipulation* and control rather than a tool for growth and responsibility. Second, banal praise following most every behavior of a child in clinic can create a feedback dependence such as that observed in children with autism who have been exposed to stimulus-response behavioral therapy (Muma & Cloud, 2010; Prizant & Wetherby, 1998). Children become reluctant to initiate communication unless prompted. It also has the potential of turning them into *praise junkies* who fail to learn to judge their own responses in the absence of comments such as "Good job!" Third, SLP-As must consider whether responses such as this are fostering independent thought or merely directing the child in how they should feel. The responsibility for determining which behaviors are, and are not, successful is shifted from the child to his teacher. Ryan remembers visiting with his professor after class and being told something to the effect of the exclamation "Hot Damn, I was on today. I couldn't have been any better!" From Ryan's perspective the class had created a fair amount of confusion. The professor's judgment certainly altered Ryan's intentions to seek clarification. Kohn suggests that the response of "Good job!" functions as *stealing a child's pleasure* by telling them how to feel rather than supporting their ability to recognize and rejoice in what they have decided is a job well done.

Kohn (1993, 2001) also suggests that with time, praise and rewards lead to a *reduction of interest* in learning skills and doing new tasks. Most clinicians working with struggling readers have observed children who, when asked what they will read over the summer, reply something to the effect of, "Why would I read anything? I'm not getting grades/points/credit for it." Critics of reading programs governed by rewards other than opportunities for continued reading have shown that such programs do not motivate children to read once the reward is achieved (Marinak, 2004). There is a common sense element to this reaction to misguided rewards, when the activity itself is not valued. Few of us enjoy engaging in long-term activities where there is little intrinsic social worth. Ultimately, Kohn (2001) states that praise such as "Good Job!" leads to a *reduction in achievement.* He argues that when the judgment of performance depends on accuracy, both engagement and risk taking are often unintentionally reduced.

Lest we paint a picture of Kohn as an advocate of cold, unemotional interactions with children, we should note that his alternative to hackneyed praise is consistent with the active constructive responding we described in Chapter 2. For example, clinicians could provide interested commenting on the qualities of what the child has done (e.g., "Sounds like you had a super summer vacation" versus "Good job talking about summer vacation."); or better yet, comments encouraging the child to let you know how they feel about their work (e.g., "What do you think about your story?" or "What was your favorite part about working with your group on the activity?"). Furthermore, Kohn writes that we empower children more if we can get them to see the impact that their performance has on others (e.g., "How did your friend respond when you shared your toys with him?" or "Did you notice how your friends giggled when you read the funny part of your story in the author's chair?"). It is the constructive responses and reactions that communication

---

**Box 5–2. Constructive Responses and
Positive Psychology**

Sometimes it is challenging to know just how often we should try to respond positively. Smith (1998) indicates that we should either respond positively to children's performance or say, "Let me show you how it is done" by modeling the desired behavior in context. In Chapter 2 Frederickson and Losada (2005) suggested that a positive dynamic relationship between positive and negative comments for enhancing adult interactions requires a ratio of 3:1, that is, three positive comments for every negative comment, with a maximum ratio of 12:1. Lidcombe suggests a 5:1 ratio, that is, five positive comments for each "corrective" response to stuttering. It is reasonable to believe that other children would benefit from such an approach. For kids in trouble, this proportion seems a bit thin; a 7:1 ratio is more likely to provide maximal benefit.

In Chapter 3, Gable and colleagues (2004) showed that only active constructive responding fosters positive relationships. ("Uh-huh" responses do not count!) Parents' "corrective" responses to their children should be "constructive" as well.

---

counselors provide that equate to the loud skills and ultimately more productive counseling.

### Creating and Using Stories

Culatta's (1994) work built on a rationale similar to that of Paley's work (1994a,b). We consider Culatta's approach and those like hers to reflect the loud technical skills. This is because the communication counselor plays an active role in determining the interaction and how it unfolds. Culatta suggests using both representational play and the re-enactment of children's storybooks as mechanisms for developing communicative competence and positive self-image in children with communication impairments. In representational play contexts, clinicians select a theme and present it to the child as the vehicle through which clinical interactions will be delivered. The clinician then collaborates with the child to create a script for the interaction (e.g., the clinician might suggest, "Let's pretend we are going to the park. What should we do when we get there?"). The clinician can then work with the child to develop and discuss possible components of the events or possible problems that could occur (e.g., "What will we do if it starts to rain?"). Props can be found or constructed (e.g., "This placemat could be our umbrella," or "Lets draw and cut out pictures that can be our food."). As the clinician and child interact, the clinician tries to make sense of, and be accepting of, all of the child's contributions. This does not mean that disagreements cannot occur. On the contrary, the clinician accepts the child's ideas as a joint communicative partner. For example, if the clinician wanted to go down the slide first upon arriving at the park and the child would rather swing, acceptance of the child's communicative contribution would involve negotiation over who gets to have their way. The therapeutic impact of this imagined play interaction comes as the clinician strategically invites the child to discuss, reflect, comment on, predict, and assess as the play unfolds. The representational play activity then functions as a format of language acquisition and narrative development (Bruner, 1983). Communication counselors ensure that the child flourishes in these interactions by promoting positive relationships and engagement.

Additionally, Culatta suggests story re-enactment as a mechanism both for narrative and for overall communicative growth. Communication counselors can select books relevant to the children's needs that are interesting, well written, and engaging to use as scripts for re-enactment. The book is shared with the child or group of children and then they are invited to act out the story with the clinician. As the clinician reads the story aloud, cloze techniques and intonation fluctuations are used to invite the child to participate in verbally producing elements of the story as they re-enact the events. Props can be created in the same ways as representational play techniques. Through the re-enactment of stories, children develop literacy skills, language proficiency, and experience motivating situations where they are successful contributors to a positive social interaction. For many of the children served by SLP-As such positive literacy experiences may be few and far between. Story re-enactments can foster a sense of optimism and willingness to persist amid barriers that arise in the process of acquiring literacy proficiency.

## Box 5–3. Connecting Children's Interests and Knowledge with Academic Structures

When Ryan was providing SLP services in a preschool classroom for children with moderate to severe impairments, there was a problem in engaging the children more fully in classroom routines so that they would be better prepared for the demands of kindergarten. Each morning the talented teacher and her classroom assistant attempted to gather the children for circle time. Ryan joined the group three mornings a week to provide services to the children on his caseload. During circle time, a review of the weather, calendar, day's activities, and a book would be shared. On a rotating basis, each day one of the children (with adult support), regardless of level of impairment, would take the role of teacher and lead the class through the routine business up to the point of the book reading; however, after several weeks the children were simply not engaging at the level we all believed they were capable. Circle time felt more like redirection time and it was certainly not productive, engaging, or fun.

One morning after another circle-time flop, the three educators were discussing what could be done. Ben, one of the higher functioning children, was enamored with a computer game that incorporated a then-popular television show "Blues Clues." In this show, an animated dog, Blue, leaves three paw-print "clues" for the human actor host to follow in order to solve a mystery of what Blue wants or where she is. Over the course of the episode, the host finds the clues, writes/draws the clue in his notebook, and once all the clues are found, sits in his "Thinking Chair" to put all of the clues together. This show was a favorite of all of the children in the room. Ben, however, was the biggest fan and would always try to sneak away from the circle to go and play the game. This particular morning, he had descended into a tantrum over not getting to play the game. As the adults talked, Ryan said, "It is a shame we can't use that game to get Ben involved in circle time." That was when the classroom teacher had what turned out to be a very wonderful idea. She responded with, "Maybe we can!"

The next day, when it was time for circle time, a laminated, blue paw print was on the ground where the child leading the group normally stood. Once this was pointed out to the children, Ben quickly identified it as a "Blues Clue." The teacher then asked the children what should be done with the clue. They all knew that clues should be written in their notebooks, so notebooks fashioned from pieces of stapled-together scrap paper were handed out along with crayons. The children were encouraged to write as best they could the picture of the clue in their notebooks. This equated to scribbling or a series of circles for most of the children; however, because the aim was to engage the children in learning to better participate in circle time, their written attempts were valued as fabulous representations of the clue. The teacher then moved the laminated paw print to the other parts of circle time using it as a device to guide the children through the activities. The game was adapted so that once the clue was written, the children would sit in their "thinking chair" spot and figure out what the clue was telling them should happen or be discussed. The children were hooked! Each day they anticipated the appearance of the first clue. After several days, a few of them began getting their notebooks and crayons ready as soon as they came into the room.

After a few weeks, another child became interested in "Dora The Explorer." So we helped the children create their own maps so that, just like Dora, they could know how to get to the places they needed to go at school. This involved two places, the cafeteria and the physical education room. While Magellan might not value these navigational devices, as communication counselors, we recognized their empowering utility for engaging the children and giving them a shared sense of control.

- How did these activities meet the intent of communication counseling?
- What quiet skills do you imagine were necessary in making these activities successful?
- What loud skills do you imagine were necessary for success?

## Counseling in Cooperative Learning Groups

Communication counselors working with children in educational settings can capitalize on strengths, build support networks, and foster resilience through the use of cooperative learning principles. Cooperative learning has a long, successful history with children who have special needs (Johnson, 2003; Johnson & Johnson, 2009). Academic and social benefits are achieved when typically developing children are grouped and collaborate with children with impairment (Harvey & Daniels, 2009; Johnson & Johnson, 1982). Heterogeneous groups, based on ability, benefit all those involved. Johnson and Johnson (2009) describe two types of cooperative learning, both of which can be easily incorporated by SLP-As into the day-to-day interactions with children. From these groups, counseling moments will arise and opportunities to value the child and build upon his or her strengths can be seized in empowering ways. Box 5–4 presents an example of how this can be accomplished with children. SLP-As can incorporate formal and informal cooperative learning techniques into their communication counseling as they seek to recognize and develop the strengths of children. Box 5–5 provides a scenario of how a child's strengths can be recognized and developed. This illustration can easily be applied to cooperative learning groups, but it requires both formal and informal techniques.

### *Formal Cooperative Learning Techniques*

Formal cooperative learning techniques are typically applied to groups of children who will be together for some extended period of time. How long a group is maintained depends on the activities and needs of the setting, but it could be anywhere from one class period, to several weeks, or even a school year. Johnson and Johnson (1999) advocate heterogeneous (based on ability) groups of three to four children. Formal cooperative learning often involves five general aspects: (a) preinstructional decision making; (b) explaining; and (c) providing tools for how instructional tasks will be accomplished and the way the cooperation will be structured; (d) monitoring how students work together and use the targeted interpersonal tools; and (e) assessing learning and how the groups and individual children function.

**Box 5–4. Identifying What Energizes and
Excites Versus Depletes and Weakens**

Positive relationships, therapeutic themes, and counseling moments can arise from collaborative activities designed to help children better understand their own motivations. Children can be encouraged to develop their communication competency by using the concepts that energize them. Strategies can be developed to manage situations more productively when they feel depleted. This activity can be adapted and completed individually, in small groups, or in classroom settings.

- Begin by identifying a child's favorite superhero, cartoon, or other fictional character.
- Collaboratively generate a list of what motivates, energizes, or excites the character.
- Make another list describing what depletes or weakens the character.
- Discuss with the child the idea that everyone is motivated, energized, or weakened in similar ways.
- Have the child create a self-portrait representing attributes from his or her list. Portraits can be created using poster board, markers, glue, scissors, magazines, or photos. (iPad apps or computer programs allow portraits to be constructed and shared electronically.)
- Communication counselors can help the child share their self-portraits with others.

SLP-As can generate thematic units from the child's list of what motivates them. For example, if the child is motivated by Legos, communication counselors can work to help the child to understand what it is about Legos that they enjoy. The child can be given the opportunity to play with Legos as a part of the therapy session where these ideas are highlighted. Perhaps a thematic unit on the history of Legos could be introduced. The child could learn about how Legos are made or the different types of Lego products. Additionally, online information can be accessed and with parental permission the child could join the online Lego Club. Communication counselors could facilitate the child's interactions with peers who share similar interests.

## Box 5–5. Developing and Using Strengths

Read the following scenario and think about ways to use the child's strengths:

Jack was struggling to fit into his new third grade classroom and to make friends. He frequently wanted to stay home from school and frequently stayed in the classroom during recess because he did not have anyone with which to play. His diagnosis of specific language impairment contributed to his academic struggles in the classroom. One of the strategies his teacher, the SLP providing services in the classroom, and his parents recognized was that they needed to find a role that would help Jack better connect with children in the classroom. Jack's parents recognized that he was creative and really liked art. Using this information, the educators decided to see if Jack would like to be the classroom photographer. He jumped at the chance. They allowed him to use the classroom's relatively inexpensive digital camera and discussed with him the types of pictures he might take.

■ What could Jack photograph that would lead to the development of his strengths and greater inclusion?
■ How can this scenario be expanded?

Perhaps Jack could be directed to photograph situations where children are working together, getting along, or some other positive interactions. Time can be built into the classroom schedule to share and discuss the photos. These photos could be used as ideas for writing projects or as reflection and review of information and activities. Having Jack identify why he took a specific picture creates opportunities for communication counselors to better understand what he attends to and believes contributes to positive interactions.

Communication counselors using cooperative learning can plan the types of activities to be performed with specific children in mind. Carefully constructed groups can allow children to not only improve their academic skills but also to enhance understanding and empathy toward others. Such groups foster acceptance, friendships, and a sense of belonging to a community. SLP-As know that these relationship connections are too often lacking with many of our children. For example, if a child with a language impairment needs a little longer to process information, or the reluctant child with a fluency disorder needs a communicative partner willing to allow him or her a chance to use their communicative strategies, a more patient and empathetic child can be identified during planning and placed in the group. Roles can be determined beforehand that play to the strengths of each group. Formal cooperative learning techniques allow for explanation of expectations and of the strategies that are to be used in the groups to ensure that everyone is allowed to fulfill their role. They also provide an opportunity for educating members of the group about one another's communication disorder. In the next chapter we discuss this form of counseling as addressing background and foreground issues in relationship to persons with aphasia. Practically speaking, from our experience it is often in the classroom or small group setting that SLP-As working with children are best able to address these issues. For instance, we can inform and address concerns children might have regarding working with a child with autism. "What is autism?" "Why does Matthew have autism?" "Can I catch autism by working with Matthew?" "Why does he not answer me when I invite him to play?" "How can I get him to play with me?" Questions such as these can be presented and discussed either by the SLP-A or by the child (if they are comfortable with and capable of doing it). Strategies and tools for interacting productively and completing cooperative learning activities can then be taught.

When cooperative learning groups are created and used over a period of time, it is important to determine ahead of time how the functioning of the groups will be monitored and what will be considered as a successful group effort. For communication counselors, successful interaction with each group member playing an important role is often sufficient. Harvey and Daniels (2009) emphasize the importance of creating and monitoring a sense of mutual interdependence among group members. Children need to learn how to value the contribution of each member. SLP-As can use their clinical interaction skills to help accomplish this by modeling the desired interactive behaviors and by mediating and coaching the children as they interact. For instance, if we consider Jack's strength of photography from Box 5–5, he could be the person responsible for providing visuals for a group report. SLP-As can support both Jack and the group as his photos are selected, presented, and explained. The group's project can be evaluated based on their success in working together and individually on how well they each performed their assigned responsibility. As the communication counselor mediates each child's interaction within the group, an appreciation for each other can develop.

Communication counselors can work with teachers to ensure that a child's strengths as applied in cooperative learning groups are included as a part of the overall assessment for the class. They can establish assessments that give voices to children about what should be included in them. Portfolios are often ideal for accomplishing this aim. For example, Kratcoski (1998) describes how the mechanics of collecting the work that comprises portfolios can provide clues for assessment. The key is that the service providers, teacher, parents, and child all determine ahead of time what work will go into the portfolio, when it will be collected, who will be responsible for it, and how the work will be assessed. Based on our experience, too often classroom portfolios consist primarily of graded worksheets or final drafts of reports. These products, while sometimes appropriate, are often not representative of the ways in which children grow and develop. The pragmatic nuances that reflect increased competency in a child's interactions with their peers are not captured in these forms. Audio or video recordings are often better at representing growth in the areas in which our clients improve; thus, they are a legitimate part of assessment of the success of cooperative learning without doubt, but incorporating media requires both planning and monitoring. Application of the five aspects of formal cooperative learning groups can create opportunities and work products that fit well into the structure of portfolios and are capable of capturing how a child changes over time.

### Informal Cooperative Techniques

Informal cooperative learning techniques can be very useful when working with children with communication disorders. These techniques are often used when children are grouped together for

---

**Box 5–6. Helping Children Identify
Strengths from Cooperative Learning Groups**

Communication counselors can assist a child in identifying his or her strengths as they are employed and developed in cooperative learning groups. The child can then be guided to determine which work products, audio or video recordings, or other materials represent those specific strengths. The child can be guided to determine how to evaluate his or her work. Written drafts and final reports, as well as recordings of interactions or performances, can be reviewed in cooperative groups or in one-on-one sessions with the SLP-A and the child. Communication counselors can help the child ask and answer questions such as:

■ What part of the cooperative group was the most interesting to me?
■ What was the best aspect of my contribution to the group?
■ Which of my strengths was most on display in the interactions?
■ What could have gone better? What would I like to change in my next group activity?
■ Did I observe strengths in others that I have or want to cultivate?
■ How was I able to support the group?
■ Was there anything that surprised me about my participation?

---

short periods of time (e.g., 3–5 min). Informal cooperative learning opportunities arise at the introduction of activities and can be created intermittently or at the conclusion of activities to reevaluate or review the child's work. For example, a child who struggles with processing multistep instructions can be paired at the beginning of an assignment with a child nearby to review directions and expectations prior starting work on the project. This same child can be provided with an opportunity to share their work with a different child at intermittent periods during the assignment. This can create opportunities for reevaluation of direction and feedback and reflection on their progress toward completion. As the project ends, the child can be grouped with others to review what the assignment was and how it was completed.

Informal cooperative learning techniques allow communication counselors flexibility to improvise and take advantage of circumstances that arise that address the needs of specific children. SLP-As can monitor the interaction and work of children in different groups for behaviors that will be of benefit to others. Once these behaviors are identified, they can create opportunities for sharing. For example, suppose Benjamin, who struggles with reading and interpretation of humor, is reading a book of knock-knock jokes to Kyle and suddenly gets the joke and reads it with the right timing and can hardly contain his excitement and laughter. A communication counselor can seize this informal opportunity and give him the chance to read the same joke to another child and then (perhaps) to the entire class.

Other informal cooperative learning opportunities can empower children by allowing them to function as the experts. If Sarah has already completed an assignment or looked up the information needed in a report, she can be invited to share that information or how she found it with others. These interactions need not take long and do not usually involve a lot of advanced preparation on the part of the communication counselor, but they can have a profound impact on a child's sense of self-worth and community. These opportunities give children a chance to share their success and foster healthy interpersonal relationships where their strengths are displayed. Positive psychology's focus on what is "right" in life can be highlighted and enhanced.

## Helping Children with Communication Disorders to Feel "Right" About Themselves

The following 10 starting points, presented in no specific order of importance, are illustrative activities based on positive psychology exercises and adapted for use with Billy, a 10- to 12-year-old boy who has a communication disorder. All activities can be in written or spoken form, but importantly, they also must be discussed. Note that they do not address the communication disorder, although it should not be denied, but the counselor should discourage Billy from focusing the activities on it. They can be effectively used as topics for small group discussions with Billy and other children of similar age. These activities are suggested as adjuncts for other therapies, not as substitutes for them. With appropriate adjustments, most of these activities are equally applicable to other ages as well.

1. Billy could be encouraged to complete the child version of the Values in Action measure (VIA) suggested in Chapter 2 (available at http://www.authentichappiness.org). Discuss the outcomes, and emphasize and exemplify the importance of knowing his strengths and of figuring out how to use them. Which ones is Billy sad about *not* having? What can he do about it? How can Billy use the strengths to leverage the not-so-strong points? Help Billy to understand the difference between not-strengths and weaknesses. Suggest that he use one of his signature strengths every day for a week, and report the results.

2. Find out who Billy's heroes are. What are their strengths? Why are they appealing? How can they become a metaphor? (Metaphor is a word for counselors, not Billy.) How can they be helpful to Billy in solving problems? For example, if Spider Man were being bullied, what would he do? Or Captain Underpants, if he was facing these problems?[4]

3. Ask Billy to tell a story about his happiest day this year. What was so good about it? It did not "just happen." What part did Billy play in making it so good?

4. Ask Billy to tell a story about something he did that made him very proud. What strengths did it show? Why is it good to be proud of oneself?

5. Ask Billy to tell three really good things about his parents, his siblings, or other people that he likes. When he goes home tonight, he is to thank his parents and siblings for them and report back.

6. If Billy has a bad day, help him to analyze why, looking out for the "thinking traps" mentioned in Chapter 2, with an extended analysis and application provided in Chapter 8). His bad days may be related largely to his communication disorder. When

---

[4]Dav Pilkey, who invented Captain Underpants, is a hero of mine. According to his website (http://www.pilkey.com), he grew up with LLD and later capitalized on his drawing skills to develop a loony and outrageous collection of childhood fantasy stories for kids that embody many principles of positive psychology.

this is so, help him to remember that his communication is not the only thing. Do not focus on the communication disorder—help him to dispute it and refute it.

7. Ask Billy to think of three good things that happened to him yesterday. How did he cause them to happen?

8. Talk to Billy about a person who has really been good to him. What did this person do? Have Billy figure out a short thank-you speech for this person, deliver it, and report back.

9. Ask Billy to choose a good friend, and list four reasons why he likes this person. Have Billy tell his friend.

10. What nice things does Ms. X (Billy's teacher) do? Billy's assignment is to thank her next time she does something nice, either for the class or for Billy himself.

These suggestions for simple but often highly effective interventions are based on understanding of communication disorders and their counseling, and on some awareness of developments in the field of positive psychology. Specific counseling issues for children with communication disorders can be addressed using a proactive approach. They include the following:

- *Self-advocacy.* Ylvisaker and Feeney (1998) urge the preparation of self-advocacy tapes, a practice in which Billy prepares a videotape that his teachers and other helping professionals can watch to help them understand him.

- *Handling teasing and bullying.* Teasing and bullying probably are universal burdens for those who are different. Communication counselors can ensure that schools have effective bully-prevention programs in place. They can foster a sense of understanding and mutual respect through skillful use of collaborative learning interactions. The clinician can also ensure that Billy understands how to access support through the school's plan.

- *Setting tolerance levels for teasing: tattletale versus silent victim.* Gladwell (2005) noted that one of childhood's most difficult lessons is learning the ins and outs of being a tattletale. This probably is particularly hard for children with disabilities as they deal with their insensitive peers. Have Billy work on how to handle telling on teasers and bullies: When is it right to tell the teacher? What level or amount of teasing demands it? What does not? What are the advantages and disadvantages of telling and not telling?

- *Laughing lessons.* The healing power of laughter seems to be considerably underplayed in relationship to challenges. Learning not only when but how to lighten up and how to help others to laugh are both skills that can be useful to children with communication disorders. Two examples follow:

  a. Helping children to differentiate the big problems from the little ones, and the intermediate ones, is a proactive skill. To this end, create or discuss a series of mishaps or scenarios, some of which include the specific challenges confronting him. Have Billy evaluate the calamity factor of each, provide a solution, and determine if there is anything to laugh about in the mishap. A few possible scenarios follow:

     - You get mud on your new sneakers the very first time you wear them
     - You forget to defrost the hamburger that you promised your mother you would defrost
     - You punch your sister when she calls you a dummy
     - The family cat knocked over a box of cereal, and because you were seen cleaning it up, your dad yells at you for spilling it.

  b. Have Billy consult a joke book and find three jokes that he thinks are funny. Have him tell the jokes to five people and evaluate their reactions.

- *Education of peers and self-disclosure: speaking/writing about the communication disorder.* In cooperation with his teacher, work with Billy and the class to prepare a short speech on their challenges to present to each other in the class. The rationale for this activity is as follows: Helping classmates to understand each other's challenges can help to allay any discomfort about them, thereby lessening the impetus for teasing. It also diverts focus from the one person's challenges, and open acknowledgement and appeals for support can undercut reasons for teasing and create positive alliances with compassionate children. They can be encouraged to ask classmates what they have learned from each other's presentations.

■ *Resilience training.* Approaches to resilience training for children have become available recently and are easily accessible to parents and clinicians via http://www.reflective learning .com, as discussed in Chapters 2 and 8. Consider ways in which you can incorporate such training into the management of children with both early-onset and later-onset disorders.

## Addressing Children Who Over- and Underestimate Their Abilities

We have acknowledged and advocated for embracing children where they currently are and not defining them by their diagnostic label. We have stated that communication counselors must empower children by, to the extent possible, accepting their communication attempts and focusing on the intention that underlies those attempts. We should assume that the child is attempting to do the very best they can and we should embrace that; however, we are not "Pollyannaish" about the legitimate struggles of the children we serve. To this end, we also recognize that there are times when, because of the nature of their communication disorder, children are not the best judges of their own abilities. Often children with limited proficiency overestimate their abilities. This can lead to counseling moments that can seriously challenge our best efforts. We recognize that much is learned through taking risks, failing, and learning from those mistakes the next time we take a risk. In this way failure can be a powerfully effective teacher. The key for communication counselors is to make sure that children are supported and valued as they take risks, and that we help them develop understanding of both their successes and failures.

## Communication Counseling with Children Who Have Communication Disorders: PERMA Considerations

In Chapter 2 we reviewed the tenets of positive psychology and signature strengths as identified through VIA assessment. At the conclusion of Chapter 4 we extended PERMA to parents of children with communication disorders. We close this chapter by reviewing the application of what we have presented here from that perspective. Application of PERMA in counseling children with communication disorders can and should take many forms. As communication counselors work with children to help prevent, diagnose, and remediate communication disorders, we can weave these principles into our interactions.

## P: Positive Affect

From a strengths-based perspective, we need to help children see what is right and positive in their lives and learn how to appreciate the value of changes that occur. By the time a child is placed on the caseload, they have usually experienced a great deal of frustration and failure. Too frequently, the bulk of responsibility for lack of success is localized within the child and does not consider if their background or life circumstances were just ill-suited for the interactional demands. For example, the child with no books in his or her home who takes longer to learn to read than others is viewed as impaired rather than impoverished, and the positive growth they make in learning is minimized by the length of time it takes.

Celebrating small but very significant positive changes can be highlighted for a child, especially in environments where these qualitative changes might be overlooked. Furthermore, communication counselors can acknowledge and help the child recognize things that they are doing well and the progress they have made.

## E: Engagement (Absorption, Immersion, Flow)

In the context of counseling children, we help them understand the importance of finding moments for engagement. This requires flexibility and a willingness to go "off script" at times. If children are productively engaged and taking appropriate risks, we can consider if our therapy plan can allow them to stay in the moment. The rejuvenating power of flow can be recognized and understood by children. When they exclaim at the end of productive time with using their strengths, "It is time to go already? It seems like we just got here!" We can help them recognize which strengths they were experiencing. We can come to know their strengths, what motivates them, and ensure that these elements are the focus of our work with them.

### R: Relationships (Involvement with Others, Sharing, Kindness, Being There)

We have described the communication counselor's responsibility for knowing what community resources are available. Furthermore, one of the major benefits of parent support groups is the opportunity they afford for the development of relationships. SLP-As can help parents recognize and accentuate VIA signature strengths in the relationships that they have. As we come to know a parent's story, we should be able to help them identify relationships where they might grow their strengths and virtues. We can then better mediate these attributes when parents experience potential misinterpretations of messages. Communication counselors functioning as models of how to reframe negative interactions and individuals willing to take time to allow parents opportunities to share can facilitate flourishing relationships.

### M: Meaning (Belonging to or Serving Something Bigger Than Oneself)

In working with children, the themes of meaning that were presented in Chapter 2 have direct application. Communication counselors can assist children in identifying and reflecting on what brings meaning to their life. Is there any way upon which similar elements could be expanded? Are there other children or cooperative learning opportunities that can allow the child to build upon these strengths? Are there ways the child can provide meaningful service to others that will allow them to feel valued? For example, can the child be given a role or assignment that allows them to connect with the group? The scenario of Jack as the photographer is one example of how this can be accomplished.

A sense of belonging and meaning can be fostered as the communication counselor helps others better understand the behaviors and motivations of children. Are there individuals who consistently misinterpret the behaviors of a child? Sometimes our best counseling efforts come through educating others and modifying the context for the child. When understanding and appropriate expectations are in place, flourishing relationships can develop.

## A: Accomplishment (Pursuing and Achieving a Goal for Its Own Sake)

The strategies we have discussed for discovering a child's story from their perspective is vital for SLP-As to provide counsel in this area. Creating interactional opportunities for a child to share his or her story can lead to major accomplishments and improved communication competence from the perspective of the child and others. Being careful in our responses to children can help them develop a capacity to gage their sense of accomplishment. When we give the child a chance to use strategies in settings that are relevant from their perspective, he or she can feel the thrill of competence as they negotiate and monitor their interactions. External reward systems are often not necessary in such situations as the successfulness of the interaction is motivation enough for continued engagement. The child who feels connected with the main character and enjoys discovering the resolution to the mystery he or she has been reading is often eager to start the next book in the series.

## Conclusion

We have provided strategies for how SLP-As can adopt a wellness perspective in the communication counseling for children with communication disorders. Hopefully we have given you ideas that can be adapted to the specific circumstances of your clinical practice. We all have signature strengths that help us find satisfaction in life. Children also have strengths that can be identified, developed, and enhanced. As you consider specific children, what might you guess are their signature strengths (see again the list in Chapter 2)? What is another way you could have helped them use that specific strength in a recent counseling moment? In the next chapter we address adults with communication disorders. Which of the strategies considered here do you think apply to adults?

# References

Bruner, J. (1983). *Child's talk. Learning to use language.* New York, NY: W. W. Norton.

Cambourne, B. (1988). *The whole story: Natural learning and the acquisition of literacy in the classroom.* Auckland, NZ: Ashton Scholastic.

Culatta, B. (1994). Representational play and story enactments: Formats for language intervention. In J. Duchan, L. Hewitt, & R. Sonnenmeier (Eds.), *Pragmatics: From theory to practice.* (pp. 105–119). Englewood Cliffs, NJ: Prentice-Hall.

Damico, J. S., Abendroth, K., Nelson, R. L., Lynch, K. E., & Damico, H. L. (2011). Research report: Variations on the theme of avoidance as compensations during unsuccessful reading performance. *Clinical Linguistics and Phonetics, 25,* 741–752.

Damico, J. S., & Damico, S. K. (1997). The establishment of a dominant interpretive framework in language intervention. *Language, Speech, and Hearing Services in Schools, 28,* 288–296.

Damico, J. S., & Nelson, R. (2005). Interpreting problematic behavior: Systematic compensatory adaptations as emergent phenomena in autism. *Clinical Linguistics and Phonetics, 19,* 405–428.

Damico, J., Nelson, R., Damico, H., Abendroth, K., & Scott, J. (2008). Avoidance strategies in an exceptional child during unsuccessful reading performances. *Clinical Linguistics and Phonetics, 22,* 283–291.

Egan, K. (1995). Narrative and learning. A voyage of implications. In H. McEwan & K. Egan (Eds.), *Narrative in teaching, learning, and research* (pp. 116–124). New York, NY: Teachers College Press.

Feldman, C. F. (1989). Monologue as problem-solving narrative. In K. Nelson (Ed.), *Narratives from the crib* (pp. 98–122). Cambridge, MA: Harvard University Press.

Fink, R. P. (1995). Successful dyslexics: A constructivist study of passionate interest reading. *Journal of Adolescent and Adult Literacy, 39*(4), 268–280.

Fredrickson, B. L., & Losada, M. (2005). Positive affect and the complex dynamics of human flourishing. *American Psychologist, 60,* 678–686.

Gable, S., Reis, H., Impett, E., & Asher, E. (2004). What do you do when things go right? The intrapersonal and interpersonal benefits of sharing good events. *Journal of Personality and Social Psychology, 87,* 228–245.

Gladwell, M. (2005). *Blink: The power of thinking without thinking.* New York, NY: Little, Brown and Company.

Hardcastle, V. G. (2003). The development of self. In G. D. Fireman, T. E. McVay, Jr., & O. J. Flanagan (Eds.), *Narrative and consciousness:*

*Literature, psychology, and the brain* (pp. 37–50). Oxford, UK: Oxford University Press.

Harvey, S., & Daniels, H. (2009). *Comprehension and collaboration: Inquiry circles in action.* Portsmouth, NH: Heinemann.

Herrera, C., Smith, S., Nelson, R. L., & Abendroth, K. (2009). Interpreting finger-flapping in the reading behaviors of an individual with Asperger Syndrome. *Asia-Pacific Journal of Speech, Language, and Hearing, 12,* 253–261.

Johnson, D. W. (2003). Social interdependence: The interrelationships among theory, research, and practice. *American Psychologist, 58,* 931–945.

Johnson, D. W., & Johnson, F. (2009). *Joining together: Group theory and group skills* (10th ed.). Boston, MA: Allyn & Bacon.

Johnson, D. W., & Johnson, R. T. (1982). The effects of cooperative and individualistic instruction on handicapped and nonhandicapped students. *Journal of Social Psychology, 118,* 257–268.

Johnson, D. W., & Johnson, R. T. (1999). Making cooperative learning work. *Theory Into Practice, 38,* 67–73.

Kasten, W. (1998). One learner, two paradigms: A case study of a special education student in a multiage primary classroom. *Reading and Writing Quarterly, 14,* 335–354.

Kohn, A. (1993). *Punished by rewards: The trouble with gold stars, incentive plans, A's praise, and other bribes.* Boston, MA: Houghton Mifflin.

Kohn, A. (2001). Five reasons to stop saying "Good job." *Young Children, 56,* 24–28.

Kratcoski, A. M. (1998). Guidelines for using portfolios in assessment and evaluation. *Language, Speech, and Hearing Services in Schools, 29,* 3–10.

Marinak, B. A. (2004). *The effects of reward proximity and choice of reward on reading motivation of third-grade students.* Ann Arbor, MI: UMI Dissertation Services.

McCabe, A., & Peterson, C. (1984). What makes a good story? *Journal of Psycholinguistic Research, 13*(6), 457–480.

McCabe, A., & Rollins, P. R. (1994). Assessment of preschool narrative skills. *American Journal of Speech-Language Pathology, 3,* 45–56.

Muma, J., & Cloud, S. (2010). Autism spectrum disorders: The state of the art. In J. S. Damico, N. Muller, & M. J. Ball (Eds.), *The handbook of language and speech disorders* (pp. 153–177). Oxford, UK: Blackwell.

Nelson, K. (1989). Monologue as representation of real-life experience. In K. Nelson, E. Oster, & J. Bruner (Eds.), *Narratives from the crib.* Cambridge, MA: Harvard University Press.

Nelson, K. (2003). Narrative and the emergence of a consciousness of self. In G. D. Fireman, T. E. McVay, Jr., & O. J. Flanagan (Eds.), *Narrative and consciousness. Literature, psychology, and the brain* (pp. 17–36). Oxford, UK: Oxford University Press.

Nelson, R., & Hawley, H. (2004). Inner control as an operational mechanism in attention deficit hyperactivity disorder. *Seminars in Speech and Language, 25,* 255–261.

Ochs, E. (2004). Narrative lessons. In A. Duranti (Ed.), *A companion to linguistic anthropology* (pp. 269–289). Oxford, UK: Blackwell.

Oldfather, P., Bonds, S., & Bray, T. (1994). Stalking the "fuzzy sunshine seeds": Constructivist processes for teaching constructivism in teacher education. *Teacher Education Quarterly, 21,* 5–14.

Paley, V. G. (1994a). Every child a story teller. In J. F. Duchan, L. E. Hewitt, & R. M. Sonnenmeier (Eds.), *Pragmatics: From theory to practice* (pp. 10–19). Englewood Cliffs, NJ: Prentice-Hall.

Paley, V. G. (1994b). Princess Anabella and the black girls. In A. H. Dyson & C. Genishi (Eds.), *The need for story. Cultural diversity in classroom and community* (pp. 145–154). Urbana, IL: National Council of Teachers of English.

Perkins, M. R. (2001). Compensatory strategies in SLI. *Clinical Linguistics and Phonetics, 15,* 67–71.

Perkins, M. R. (2005). Pragmatic ability and disability as emergent phenomena. *Clinical Linguistics and Phonetics, 19,* 367–377.

Potter C., & Whittaker C. (2001). *Communication enabling environments for children with autism.* London, UK: Jessica Kingsley.

Prelock, P. A. (2006). *Autism spectrum disorders. Issues in assessment and intervention.* Austin, TX: Pro-Ed.

Prizant, B. M., & Wetherby, A. M. (1998). Understanding the continuum of discrete-trial traditional behavioral to social-pragmatic, developmental approaches in communication enhancement for young children with autism/PDD. *Seminars in Speech and Language, 19,* 329–353.

Rydell, P. J. (2012). *Learning style profile for children with autism spectrum disorders* [Kindle DX version]. Retrieved from http://www.amazon.com/Learning-Children-Spectrum-Disorders-ebook/dp/B00B4GE9G0/ref=sr_1_1?ie=UTF8&qid=1359492224&sr=8-1&keywords=learning+style+profile+autism

Smith, F. (1998). *The book of learning and forgetting.* New York, NY: Teachers College Press.

Wells, G. (1999). *Dialogic inquiry. Toward a sociocultural practice and theory of education.* Cambridge, UK: Cambridge University Press.

Wells, G. (2001). The case for dialogic inquiry. In G. Wells (Ed.), *Action, talk, and text. Learning and teaching through inquiry.* New York, NY: Teachers College Press.

Ylvisaker, M., & Feeney, T. (1998). *Collaborative brain injury intervention.* San Diego, CA: Singular.

## Websites

http://www.litcircles.org

http://www.fromthemixedupfiles.com

http://www.lego.com

http://www.biausa.org

http://www.friendswhostutter.org

http://www.nsastutter.org

http://www.neuro.pmr.vcu.edu

http://www.pilkey.com

http://www.russhicks.com

http://www.stutteringhomepage.com

http://www3.fhs.usyd.edu.au/asrcwww/treatment/lidcombe.htm

http://www.fishfulthinking.com

# *Chapter 6*

# COMMUNICATION COUNSELING WITH ADULT CLIENTS AND THEIR FAMILIES FOR WHOM PROGRESSION IS TOWARD IMPROVEMENT

## Introduction

Except perhaps for stuttering treated in adulthood, and some adult-onset disorders, most adult communication disorders result from specific medical conditions. A close look at adult problems from a holistic perspective reveals two general patterns of progression that have profound implications for counseling: improvement (indicated by physical or functional recovery or stabilization, or both) and deterioration.

With disorders characterized by the first pattern, affected persons have a high probability of getting better, if only somewhat,

187

with the passage of time. With certain more or less obvious exceptions, such as metastatic brain cancer, the prognosis is never worse than when it is initially incurred. In conditions that result from brain damage involving cerebrovascular disease, the excision of a nonmalignant brain tumor, or the consequences of traumatic brain injury (TBI), a change toward the better may be termed "spontaneous recovery," which reflects both neuroplasticity and a more general healing process. For clients whose communication or swallowing disorder is secondary to conditions such as laryngectomy, a more appropriate term may be "healing." All of these conditions probably involve new learning and adaptation over time as well. Counseling clients with disorders that fit this more positive pattern is explored in this chapter.

Disorders characterized by the pattern of deterioration have an inevitably downward progression or may be fatal. Affected persons have a high likelihood of getting worse to some degree with the passage of time, despite appropriate treatment and intervention. Such disorders are the focus of Chapter 7.

An advantage of counseling adults with disorders of upward progression over counseling parents and children with communication disorders is that from the start, outcomes seem a bit more clear, even though similar crises are initially evident. It is easier to be optimistic. Furthermore, most adult disorders occur in midlife or thereafter, thereby constraining lifespan considerations. This is not meant to minimize the counseling concerns for persons whose problems occur later in life and have a somewhat more predictable course; rather, it simply underscores the reality that these disorders have different counseling priorities. Issues such as the likelihood of returning to work, altered family roles, retirement, social isolation, and lifestyle restrictions and changes now arise, in part supplementing more general issues such as safety, acceptance, and fulfillment, and the other issues discussed in Chapters 4 and 5.

Obviously, age also differentiates parent/child counseling in communication disorders from counseling with adults. Rather than working with children, and perhaps counseling parents who are likely to be from the clinician's own generation, now clinicians may be counseling adults nearer to the age of their parents or grandparents. Generational differences between counselors and clients do not necessarily present problems, but they may be dicey, particularly when counselors are younger than those whom they counsel. Counseling responsibilities to adults with these disorders also extend to older spouses and partners, and possibly grown children. For younger counselors, especially, it is essential to keep in mind that good counseling with older adults grows from a foundation of healthy respect for one's elders coupled with sound knowledge about the aging process.

This chapter highlights adult communication disorders that occur following stroke. It emphasizes aphasia, apraxia of speech, right hemisphere cognitive-communication disorders, dysphagia, and dysarthria. Stroke is the focus because it is the most common cause of this pattern of communication disorders; however, the counseling approach described here is easily applicable to adults with TBIs, speech disorders resulting from cancer of the larynx, and other adult communication disorders in which improvement over the passage of time can be comfortably assumed.

Because this chapter concerns the multiple consequences of a single type of event, it starts with a brief discussion of specific stroke features that affect communication counseling. Next it discusses communication problems that follow stroke. The varying counseling needs of persons who experience stroke and their caregivers are then related to the time course of recovery. Aphasia serves as the focus disorder.

## Stroke and Communication Counseling

What aspects of stroke in and of itself are important to communication counseling? Some issues are in the background but are likely to influence the tone of communication counseling covertly but pervasively; others are foreground questions to which counselors need to provide answers.

### Background Issues

Two broad concerns lurk in the background: First, stroke has seriously threatened the affected person's life, with implications for both that person and the spouse or family; and second, stroke changes previous goals and priorities, sometimes unavoidably. Each situation is discussed next.

- *Stroke is a brush with death, and a reminder of the transience of life, for both the person who experiences stroke and the family.* Even the term "stroke survivor" reflects the drastic nature of the event. For most people, such events—stroke, serious head injury, or detection of cancer, for example—are bound up with issues of death and dying and may serve as wake-up calls to live more fully and more wholesomely, or may lead to reaffirmation of religious faith. A stroke is frightening for persons who experience one, as well as for people around them. Fear and anxiety center on the apprehension that another stroke will occur; such feelings often are the culprits in instances of overprotection and disproportionate cautiousness. Capable communication counselors must acknowledge fear and anxiety but be prepared to supply antidotes, ranging from providing useful simple information to helping affected persons engage in activities designed to reduce their stress and distress. Chapter 8 includes such an activity, centered on the familiar concern of family members' fear of leaving their aphasic family member alone. The activity uses a model called "real-time resilience" by Reivich and Shatté (2002). It is an extremely useful approach in the group workshop format described in Chapter 8, but it is also useful for individual counseling.
- *Stroke changes reality.* Communication disorders, as well as many of stroke's other accompaniments, cause major lifestyle changes for many people. These accompaniments include new worries about finances, role changes, living arrangements, social life, leisure time, driving, and many more. At least some such factors exist for every stroke family, and each of them underscores the need for helping families to develop resilience and optimism, and to reestablish a sense of self.

## Foreground Issues

In addition to background issues, there are usually two major immediate concerns for affected persons and their families. Neither the causes nor the general effects of stroke are well known to most people. Both aspects influence recovery and require explication. Each aspect is discussed next from a counseling perspective.

■ *What is a stroke, anyway?* As noted in Chapter 1, this question seems particularly pertinent early in the recovery process. The crisis atmosphere immediately surrounding stroke often makes it difficult for patients and families to absorb even simple and accurate explanations, because they are experiencing shock and denial. Interestingly, even when the information has apparently gotten through, affected persons and families for whom the stroke is in the distant past seldom are bored by the topic and continue to listen intently as the information is presented again. This applies to family members as well as the individuals who have been directly affected. For both, hearing the general stroke facts repetitively and reiterating one's own stroke story appear to reduce fear and anxiety. Once the initial period is over, telling the story again and again also seems to emphasize the distance traveled on the road to successful management. Furthermore, revisiting the topic seems to be reassuring. Clinicians should also revisit stroke facts, as opposed to stroke stories, not only to help people understand what has happened, but to update information about latest treatments, if any changes have occurred (Box 6–1).

■ *Why did it happen to me/us?* The preferred term today is stroke, rather than cerebrovascular accident (or CVA), according to the American Stroke Association (ASA), an affiliate of the American Heart Association, as well as the National Stroke Association (NSA). Both groups object to the notion of "accident"; rather, they emphasize that stroke has known risk factors, and that prevention of stroke involves being aware of risk factors and engaging in wellness behaviors that mitigate them. Alertness to signs that a stroke is impending also is stressed. In fact, the NSA lobbies for the term "brain attack," equating it with "heart attack," to underscore the urgency of recognizing early stroke symptoms and getting help immediately.

Programs aimed at prevention are of undeniable importance. Communication counselors, however, are involved with people

> ### Box 6–1. Guidelines for Communication Counselors' Stroke Facts Presentations
>
> 1. Update information frequently.
>    a. Eliminate professional jargon.
>    b. Use diagrams.
>    c. Include risk factors and warning signs and what to do about them.
>    d. The goal is empowerment, not threat.
>    e. Provide updates about useful and informative films, YouTube presentations, and so forth.
> 2. Practice your presentation with your family or some friends.
>    a. Tell it simply and clearly.
>    b. Seek confirmation about what they understood.
>    c. Get their feedback.
>    d. Provide written materials.

who have not prevented stroke. These clients need to understand how and why it happened, perhaps to prevent a reoccurrence but perhaps also to deal with blame and guilt. How did it happen? Modifiable risk factors may have not been recognized, or perhaps the person who had the stroke did not follow physician recommendations to make lifestyle changes, or perhaps the spouse or other family members also were unaware of risks, or failed to make them clear or to support needed changes. Perhaps risk factors were attended to, and the stroke happened anyway.

In any case, guilt and anger may rule. In fact, guilt and anger often compete, and often depression raises its ugly poststroke head as well. A personal story from Audrey illustrates these dynamics:

> My husband, a neurologist and far more knowledgeable about stroke than I, suffered a stroke. As an experienced aphasiologist, I was well aware of risk factors, and I knew (as did he) that being overweight, failing to exercise, eating a questionable diet and drinking excessively were problematic. All were in play, and I was worried.
>
> Did I point all this out? Of course! Did I make a convincing case? No. I tried, unsuccessfully, or at least not in time.

Was my failure to convince him due to the possibility he was rejecting what I had to say because I was a nag? Possibly. Was it due to the fact that I made my case poorly? Also possibly.

After the stroke, how did he feel? Guilty because he knew better, for sure. And embarrassed—this should not have happened to a knowledgeable neurologist. But in for a few risk factors (not all), he subsequently changed his ways. Finally, he was angry with me for being right (as well as my being unsuccessful in suppressing "I told you so"). And he was depressed, a natural consequence of stroke.

After the stroke, where was I emotionally? I was scared. I was angry because he had not listened to me. I felt guilty because I had not made my case appropriately. I felt totally powerless. Despite the fact that my husband returned to work, did the stroke influence our relationship? You bet!

This stroke had relatively minimal physical and functional consequences, none of which involved communication. Nevertheless, those questions lingered, unanswered and unresolved, for a long time into our healing process.

This story is merely a vehicle for pointing out that a complex dynamic is likely to underlie the apparently simple question of "Why did this happen to me?" The complexity has substantial potential to influence not only counseling but the course of intervention as well.

## Accompanying Problems

It is well known that in addition to the communication problems that result from stroke, physical and cognitive effects also can complicate the counseling picture. This section summarizes some ways in which these effects interact with our counseling responsibilities.

### Mobility

Because of their focus on communication, SLP-As sometimes are rather dismissive of the burdens imposed by paralysis or paresis on persons and families. Mobility issues may serve as strong deterrents to receiving outpatient care and often contribute to family fatigue. Furthermore, hard as it may be for some of us in this profession to believe, mobility problems may be more important than communication problems for some people who have had a stroke. For example, an aphasic man from the University of Arizona Aphasia Clinic who was an avid hunter and fisherman before his stroke took his aphasia in stride, but he was devastated by his inability to pursue the outdoor life. Possibly the best thing that happened in his aphasia rehabilitation was when he and his clinician jointly researched, found, and evaluated adaptive fishing rods and handicapped-accessible fishing piers. Please also note that this example provides a good model of intertwining counseling and direct language work.

## Cognition

Cognitive problems that sometimes accompany stroke may be elusive in some cases and confounding in others. The slogan of the Adler Aphasia Center, in Maywood, New Jersey, is "Aphasia: Loss of words, not intellect." The Aphasia Center of West Texas in Midland puts the message this way: "I know more than I can say: Aphasia: a loss of language, not intelligence." Both of these messages share a viewpoint that is well engrained in SLPs, for the good reason that in most cases they are true.

When a person has incurred many strokes, however, or when stroke occurs in a person who has had previous cognitive decline, this picture may be altered. Furthermore, persons with severe global aphasia, complicated possibly by dysarthria and apraxia of speech, also have increased probability of the co-occurrence of additional neuropsychological problems such as difficulty in problem solving (Helm-Estabrooks, 2002). Moreover, in such persons, because of the extent of their language deficits, additional problems may be particularly difficult to identify and treat.

Clients with right hemisphere brain damage (RHD) also present significant challenges in this regard. First, they share the characteristics of disorganized, egocentric, pragmatically compromised, tangential, and digressive language use with dementing persons and those with TBI. "Cognitive communication disorders" is our shorthand for implying that their language has links to more extensive (if sometimes subtle) impairments. Of course, impairments such as anosognosia and neglect of the left hemispace complicate the cognitive picture for RHD people as well.[1]

Denial and anosognosia in persons with RHD require special consideration. The question, "When is a problem a problem?" can occur across the spectrum of adult communication disorders, but it is especially urgent in RHD and possibly in TBI as well. Many cognitive-communicative manifestations of RHD may be subtle and minimally apparent to casual acquaintances. Clearly, their presence is a counseling concern, and there are ethical considerations as well. No general answer is possible here, but how a "problem" is defined and who defines it as such constitute important issues for communication counselors.

### Psychiatric and Psychological Issues

According to the National Institute of Mental Health (2006), depression is estimated to have a prevalence of between 10% and 27%, increasing by 15% to 40% in the first 2 months after stroke. Depression therefore is a major concern, because when it occurs, it can impede the rehabilitation process. If depression is suspected, clinicians must bring it to the immediate attention of physicians, who may prescribe antidepressant medication. Two such drugs have been shown to be particularly effective with stroke: tricyclic antidepressants and selective serotonin reuptake inhibitors.

Although "talking therapies" have a respected role in the management of depression in general, they are often of limited use in persons with stroke-related language and speech disorders. In some instances, cotreatment conducted by a mental health specialist and an SLP can be beneficial, but this is a luxury for most people. This cotreatment is likely to include some of the exercises derived from cognitive-behavior therapy, as discussed earlier. In addition, adaptations of the resilience approaches described in Chapter 8

---

[1]The most extensive interaction among language and cognitive problems occurs with TBI, of course, as pointed out earlier, and with dementias, as described in Chapter 7. Very few adults who have incurred TBI develop stroke-like aphasia; even fewer persons with dementia do. On the contrary, in most cases the psychosocial consequences of the disorders simply manifest through language and language problems.

can be modified for use with people with aphasia and applied creatively to aphasia treatment, most likely by a cotreatment team with appropriately trained psychologists; however, the most important consideration for communications counselors regarding poststroke depression is to be alert for its signs in both affected persons and family members, and to refer appropriately if it is found. It also is essential to provide a supportive environment for poststroke clients and their families who are experiencing depression as they participate in treatment for communication disorders. The three possible sources for depression after stroke are listed in Box 6–2.

### Psychosocial Issues

Box 6–2 makes it clear that people can be depressed before a stroke or can incur depression as a consequence. Other factors also can be involved. For example, strokes can happen to people with bad marriages, nasty personalities, and decidedly unhelpful children. Stroke has seldom been known to solve such problems or to alter such circumstances favorably; rather, they become counseling issues.

Although it is not an inevitable consequence, social isolation frequently affects people who have had a stroke, particularly those with resultant aphasia. Along with other consequences of aging, the slipping away of friends and social contacts is also a particularly cruel aftermath of stroke. One of the most beneficial results of participation in stroke and aphasia groups (and spouse groups as well) is that it breaks this chain of loneliness. In many instances, deep friendships are formed and extend beyond the contacts made in groups.

A review of risk factors for stroke is appropriate here: advancing age, high blood pressure, tobacco use, diabetes, carotid artery disease, sickle cell disease, high blood levels of "bad" cholesterol

---

**Box 6–2. Sources of Depression in Stroke**

- Depression can occur as a neural accompaniment of stroke.
- Depression can occur as a reaction to stroke (in family members also, of course).
- Depression can precede the stroke (in family members also, of course).

and low levels of "good" cholesterol, obesity, physical inactivity, excessive alcohol intake, and drug use. This list of risk factors supports the notion that stroke is hardly an "equal opportunity disease." The relative prevalence rates for differing socioeconomic levels in the United States make it clear that stroke does not statistically favor America's "rich and famous." Statistical trends do not predict individual patterns and variability, but this list of risk factors suggests that many economic and social problems can accompany stroke and influence counseling of those who experience it.

In the following case example, the affected person does not fit a predictable stroke pattern, but some of the possible counseling concerns are well illustrated:

> Matt Z is an upper-middle-class, 65-year-old white man who did not smoke and who worked out regularly, ate very carefully, drank moderately, and had unremarkable findings on yearly physical examinations. He held a powerful position in a major company where he was reputed to have had fairly contentious relationships with his colleagues and subordinates. Following his retirement, Mr. Z and his wife, Clara, moved to Arizona, where he began to indulge his passion, golf. Six months later, he had a moderately severe right hemisphere stroke, with resulting significant cognitive and communicative consequences and severe left hemiplegia.
>
> Clara Z, his now bewildered and vaguely angry wife, is 15 years his junior and went to Arizona with him to play golf and to enjoy the rich social life available in their community. Mr. Z's three children from a previous marriage are somewhat concerned about him but do not seem to grasp the details of his situation, and they all live far away; moreover, their relationship with him is rather strained because they are still confused about why he divorced their mother 10 years earlier.

Here is an exercise: Examine the psychosocial features that could influence Mr. Z's recovery, even in the absence of a detailed clinical assessment of his stroke. Determine those features that play a role in counseling both husband and wife. Successful communication counselors should try to be aware of all of the factors that influence successful treatment and recovery, and they should be prepared to deal with them.

This rapid sweep through the broad territory of stroke should alert clinicians to the idea that although a specific person's speech and language profile affects the poststroke clinical course, interventions, counseling, and outcome, there are many other influences as well. Indeed, most medical problems occur in complex contexts, such as with TBI, cancer, and kidney disease. Such complexity reminds us that our goals are to treat people, not their impairments.

## Communication Problems after Stroke

This book is biased toward communication problems. This chapter is particularly biased in its insistence that communication disorders are stroke's most devastating consequence. But outside of our own profession, communication problems are likely to be stroke's most easily marginalized consequences. Why is this so?

Communication, like breathing, is pervasive and frequently is taken for granted. As a result, even most other health care professionals fail to recognize the extent to which communication problems can have profound negative effects on quality of life. Sadly, this remains true for most people until communication problems personally affect them. Families also take communication for granted and fail to recognize the potentially catastrophic effects of communication problems before they experience them.

The marginalization increases with a stroke that results in communication problems. For most lay people, talking and thinking are practically synonymous terms. Loss of ability to talk well may be construed as an indication that thinking also is compromised. Furthermore, one's identity and sense of self are muted or altered when the means to express them are limited; hence, the sage advice of the mottoes of the two centers previously mentioned.

The foregoing reflects the darker side of the stroke experience, but there is also a lighter side. Stroke is an example of the Zorba-like notion of the "full catastrophe." As borne out in our own clinical experience, the negative effect on the lives of aphasic persons and their families often can be tempered or neutralized by behaviors that are counter to what has been presented to them as immutable "stroke fact." For example, consider what happens to a spouse when the person with aphasia says her name when the doctor told her he would never talk again, or what happens to the aphasic person himself? In addition to being an occasion for celebration, it may well set the stage for continued improvement. This would not necessarily be just spontaneous recovery. What people bring to stroke and to other potentially devastating conditions is as important as what the disorders bring.

Additional support for this perspective comes from stories from other professionals and reports written by stroke persons and their families, along with websites relating to their recovery. Brief stories of persons who have brought personal strengths and unique attitudes to their recovery include the following: Roger Ross (described in Holland and Ramage, 2004) essentially neutralized his own aphasia by devoting himself to developing aphasia groups for others to attend. Mike and Elaine Adler put their energies to work to build the Adler Aphasia Center after Mike's stroke (http://www.adleraphasiacenter.org). Eileen Quann (2002) chronicled her experiences as a spouse in a way that extends her helpful hand to other stroke families. Carol Dow-Richards became a stroke advocate after her son, David, became aphasic at the age of 10 years. David himself, now in his late twenties is a co-founder, with Christine Huggins, of the Aphasia Recovery Connection, a Facebook virtual support group founded in 2012 for young people with aphasia and listed among the relevant websites. David described his own recovery in a recent book (2013). Sean Maloney, still struggling with speech as a result of a stroke in 2010, was appointed Chairman of Intel China in 2011 and has returned to competitive racing. Tommye-Karen Mayer (2000), and Paul Berger and Stephanie Mensch (1999), wrote very helpful and practical books about living with hemiplegia (and in Bergers, case aphasia). Robert McCrum (1999) chronicled his right hemisphere stroke. Actor Kirk Douglas (2003) described getting on with his life as a person with dysarthria. One amazing final example is that of Dorothea Wender (1989), a professor of classics who had an aphasia-producing stroke. Wender wrote inspiring stories of her recovery and published her own experiment on the efficacy of her self-designed and self-delivered therapy in a major neurology journal.

Not all people greet stroke or its aftermath as challenges, nor are they constitutional optimists, nor do they do heroic things or write books about their stroke experiences. Many people are simply everyday folks who live successfully with aphasia, learning to take life's setbacks in stride and serving as role models for their peers. (A number of such stroke stories can be found in the journal *Topics in Stroke Rehabilitation*, volume 13.1, 2006.) Of particular note is the extensive group of personal stories that were collected by Hinckley (2006). Box 6–3 describes one of Audrey's most moving experiences in this regard.

The good news is that counseling, coaching, all the beautiful stories that continue to proliferate on YouTube, and strong peer support all can help people who are overwhelmed, helpless, and hopeless. People can be aided to see things differently, to capitalize on their strengths, and to develop some degree of resilience as a result. This is the bright side of counseling, but one not often recognized or emphasized.

This section cannot close without reference to Diane Ackerman's (2011) marvelous book concerning the aftermath of her husband Paul West's stroke and resultant aphasia, *One Hundred Names for Love*, which should be required reading for all clinical aphasiologists. Only after the end of formal therapy that focused on West's language problems and plugging up the holes in his language did Ackerman begin to build on her husband's strengths. Their marriage, in many ways, was cemented by their love of language and the book soars with ways in which she built on their word-mongering habits—leaning, trusting, building, and playing on them. Few aphasic people have West's strengths; few families, Ackerman's insights and abilities. Nevertheless, this book lays out the universal principles involved in living fully, despite aphasia. Never has it been more clearly shown that language is not lost in aphasia but is instead scrambled, lurking and unfettered inside the person who has experienced it.

## Counseling for Aphasia, Right Hemisphere Cognitive Disorders, Dysarthria, and Apraxia of Speech: Differing Goals at Different Times

As persons with communication disorders begin their journey toward some degree of resolution, they and their clinicians both need to be reminded once again that no one knows how far along

**Box 6–3. Everyday Resilience:**
**Clinical Example**

A large group of aphasic individuals and their families had assembled for a workshop on aphasia. I was the group leader, and I knew nobody in the room except a clinician or two, and most of the families were strangers to each other as well. I began by introducing myself and telling a bit of my story, and then I suggested we go around the room and share stories with each other. My job was going to be simply to highlight important stroke facts, or aphasia truisms that the stories were revealing, particularly those that were likely to have meaning for others in the room. Not surprisingly, some people found it easy to talk; others were more reticent. Sometimes it was the person with aphasia who spoke, sometimes the spouse or caregiver, and sometimes both, and as we went along, the discussion warmed with shared experiences.

Finally, it was the turn of a man whose aphasia had almost totally resolved, and he told his story, starting with the previous day, when he retook his real estate examination and began the process of returning to work. Then he said: "But now I want to tell you something really important. I have had two events in my life that I viewed as personal disasters. The first was when I was drafted to fight in Vietnam, and the second was when I had my stroke two years ago. As I look back now, I realize that they were the most important events in my life. I hated both of them. They were both awful, but they were what I have learned the most from. They taught me what life is about and why I should cherish it. And they taught me who I am."

There was silence. I was too close to tears to attempt to break it. The ice was broken instead by a woman who had already told us that she was talking for her husband George as well as for herself because he could not talk at all. This time she said: "All I can say is thank you. I never told you this before, George, but your stroke is the most important thing that has happened to me, too. It taught me what love is."

that path anyone may travel. In counseling poststroke clients, the crystal ball is always cloudy. Not only is it unethical to pretend otherwise, but facilitating unjustifiable hope also is cruel. Nevertheless, because the poststroke clinical course progresses positively over time, some substantial recovery from aphasia, RHD, apraxia of speech, dysphagia, and dysarthria can be expected. This is particularly likely to occur with appropriate intervention (see Robey, 1998, for information on efficacy of aphasia rehabilitation, for example). Families and individuals with communication disorders must be made explicitly aware of positive change and encouraged to watch for it—not full recovery necessarily, but changes in that direction. Progression toward improvement also implies that change itself may result in differing counseling agendas at different times. Counselors must be prepared to accommodate change. Accordingly, counseling issues for three time intervals are discussed next: first at the onset of aphasia, during the acute phase; then during its rehabilitation phase; and finally, during its chronic phase. These phases and changing agendas are relevant to aphasia, dysarthria, and apraxia of speech, but for simplicity, aphasia is used here as an exemplar.

With RHD, timing of counseling to issues as they arise is not quite so simple. Specifically, unless the stroke and its consequences leave severe right hemisphere impairments, such as extensive anosognosia or hemispatial neglect, many of its communication consequences may be somewhat masked at the onset and become a concern only during rehabilitation or in chronic phases. Nevertheless, if the problems experienced early on by the client with RHD are relevant, then the counseling principles presented next are appropriate.

## Counseling at the Onset

A series of questions appropriate for these three time periods is available in a study by Avent, Glista, Wallace, Jackson, Nishioka, and Yip (2005). The questions initially were identified in work with focus groups of families. Then, additional families, persons uninformed about stroke and aphasia and SLPs, judged the relative importance of each of the questions isolated in the development study. (As discussed later, they also looked at questions that arise upon discharge from formal rehabilitation work.) The onset-phase questions judged by 90% of the families to be extremely important are presented in Box 6–4.

In effect, this list constitutes the informational agenda for communication counselors who work with stroke families. Certainly, answers should be provided, in many forms using various media, as noted in Chapter 1 and earlier in this chapter.[2]

Nevertheless, Box 6–4 questions are retrospective, that is, study participants are looking back on their remembered informational needs, not on what they were actively seeking during the earliest days of the experience. In fact, the complex psychodynamics of the early grief period probably preclude clear memories. Taking advantage of information in the early phases of crisis probably is not possible for most families; therefore, simply providing answers to those questions is not enough. Information should be supplemented by two of the other counseling activities presented in Chapter 1: receiving information that the affected person and family wish to share, and helping them to clarify their ideas and feelings. The fourth activity, providing options for changing behaviors, is premature at the onset of stroke; in fact, a particularly delicate

---

**Box 6–4. Family Member-Suggested Information Needs at Onset of Aphasia**

- What is a stroke?
- What is aphasia?
- Where can we get more information about aphasia?
- What is the best that we can expect?
- What can we do?
- What resources are available once we leave the hospital?

(From Avent et al., 2005.)

---

[2]How do *you* explain aphasia to your patients and families? It is even more foreign than stroke, and murkier to explain, as just suggested. Practice your answers. Write them. Hand them out.

counseling task is to help people understand why detailed planning probably should wait, at least for a bit. Relevant counseling activities also include simply listening to concerns about the future, sharing sadness and frustration, offering the immediate help that the clinician feels is within the scope of practice for counseling, being supportive, and holding the client's hand.

## Acute Intervention: Getting Off to a Good Start

Holland and Fridriksson (2001) have written in detail about early treatment after onset of aphasia.[3] Put briefly, their contention is that in the acute phase of stroke, clinicians should intersperse and intertwine counseling as described above, with direct intervention. In other words, communication counselors should use clinical encounters to get patients and families off to a good start. We urge the use of activities that can illustrate spontaneous recovery to patients and families, and that are embedded into the familiar medium of conversation, to emphasize what the affected person can still do in the earliest days following stroke, despite aphasia. These principles are briefly described next.

### *Illustrating Spontaneous Recovery*

Families and patients (they are still "patients" at this point in their recovery) are not well positioned to understand the language behaviors that comprise communication impairments. Talking about spontaneous recovery and change probably will not get through. Showing families and patients what is happening, rather than just telling them about it, is likely to be more effective. It is possible to illustrate for families and patients what spontaneous recovery is all about, focusing on aspects of communication that are still intact, rather than on what language is currently not retrievable.

How can we illustrate spontaneous recovery? One way is by taking note of daily changes (preferably using repetitive activities) and bringing the changes to the attention of both aphasic persons

---

[3]For an entirely different view of early treatment, see Peach 2001, and Godecke, Hird, Lalor, Rai, and Phillips (2013).

and their families. For example, the clinician may say something like: "Mr. Jones, that was great! Mrs. Jones, yesterday when I saw your husband, I asked him what your name was, and I didn't understand what he said. And today, when you walked in, he said 'Hi, Maude' clear as a bell. Did you both notice that? Mr. Jones, give yourself a pat on the back for the progress! Changes like that even have a name—'spontaneous recovery' (write it). Glad to see it's kicking in."

Rather than practicing abstract drills and such, using repetitive activities incorporated into conversation can reveal small daily changes. The goal is to capitalize on communication strengths, rather than to lay bare communication impairments.

### *Using Conversation*

The reason for embedding such tasks into conversation is that conversation is natural. Even in the earliest days after stroke, conversation encourages marginal strengths to emerge. By focusing on this natural process, clinicians can help aphasic persons and their families to mitigate the "identity theft"—Shadden's term (2005)—that results when adults develop communication disorders. Shadden also notes that although clinicians always believe they support their client's sense of competency, "we use labels that point to incompetence, and recognize our clients for their impairment" (p. 219). Our clinical tasks often also highlight impairment; therefore, particularly in the very early phases after stroke, it is crucial to highlight what is right, rather than what is wrong. Clinicians should focus on preserved behaviors, and do it in the most natural way, by encouraging talking and conversation.

### *Activities for Acute Treatment*

The foregoing has been a brief summary of the approach detailed by Holland and Fridriksson (2001). Many additional suggestions for activities are provided there. Box 6–5 samples some that are consistent with this approach to early management. Some of the activities are designed to involve families and thus aimed at answering the question raised by Avent and colleagues (2005) about what families can do to help; others are suggestions for clinicians.

### Box 6–5. Suggested Activities for Poststroke Clients and Families

The case of Mrs. M, who suffered a stroke two days previously and has aphasia, is used as an example.

Activities for family members:

- Explain that keeping track of what Mrs. M says, and how well she seems to understand, would be very useful. Provide a small notebook and a pencil, and ask family members to record what was said, when, and a very brief summary of the circumstances. Give examples, and ask them to leave the notebook in the room for your use when you come in each day. Also, use the notebook to communicate back to them.
- Ask family to write a brief "story" of Mrs. M, that is, her work and interests, some things about the family and other significant people, family member names, some likes and pet peeves, TV habits, and so on. Instead of a story, you might develop a form for families to fill in. Either way, it will help you and other health care professionals to make treatment materials relevant.

Activities for clients/acute care clinicians:

- *Comprehension*: Fill in the menu form together; ask Mrs. M some relevant questions that you know the answers to (perhaps from the brief story above); provide sequential commands involving objects in the room. Use Mrs. M's responses as the basis for charting. Provide feedback concerning appropriateness and differences from previous day.
- *Reading*: Read get-well cards, daily schedules, or menus together; check for amount of support required. As with comprehension activities, keep track of Mrs. M's responses for her chart, and provide feedback.
- *Spoken language*: Check family names; watch some TV together and ask questions about what is happening; hold relevant simple conversations. As for other com-

ponents of monitoring, track Mrs. M's responses and provide feedback.

- *Speech production*: Note changes in dysarthria or apraxia of speech in Mrs. M's speech; track and provide feedback.
- *Swallowing*: The centerpiece of acute care: If the clinician is feeding or observing Mrs. M during meals, it is the best time to practice conversation as well (between careful chewing, chin tucks, and other self-protection maneuvers), and also check on comprehension.

(Modified from Holland & Fridriksson, 2001.)

## Documenting and Data

It is important to keep careful track of daily changes and improvements. They become part of the progress notes, but they also should be shared with families, patients, and other staff members. Such documentation is the written record of spontaneous recovery and behavioral strengths.

Holland and Fridriksson (2001) formalized the approach just described and analyzed data to support its effectiveness when acute care stays lasted longer than a week.[4] There is now considerably more urgency concerning how to provide counseling in the constrained time frame that characterizes present lengths of hospital stay. One goal is answering the important questions, but the other is getting off to a good start. To enter a rehabilitation center with a little of one's self-esteem and self-efficacy intact is a tremendous boost to recovery.

## Moving to Rehabilitation

People should now lose their "patient" (i.e., helpless) designation. Health care professionals appear to expect that people will improve significantly if they work hard enough in rehabilitation. SLPs now

---

[4]That was not during the First World War—it was about 1990!

abet the "good start" with the "power of therapy." Another subtle message comes with this one: rehabilitation is where the recovery action is. This is partially true, but to maximize it, and to prepare for the future, there are two additional early tasks for communication counselors. One task concerns the expectations of affected persons and their families about rehabilitation: "dispelling rehabilitation magic." The other task concerns learning the rehabilitation ropes: "solving the rehabilitation mystery." In what follows, counseling involves not only a set of tools but also a specific attitude. This is not an accident; it feels contextually appropriate to the fast pace of rehabilitation. ("Counseling moments" have not been abandoned; they are picked up by the boxful later in this chapter.)

### *Expectations: Dispelling Rehabilitation Magic*

At the onset of aphasia (see Box 6–4), families have already asked, "What is the best we can expect?" (Avent et al., 2005). This question still looms large at the beginning of rehabilitation. Not only is the question scary for families and people with aphasia and TBI and RHD, but it also constitutes a challenge for clinicians because it puts them on the tightrope between offering false hope and projecting Eeyore-type gloom and doom. The question requires an answer. It demands forthrightness about saying, "I don't know" while simultaneously acknowledging the importance of hope and the need to be optimistic.

Many rehabilitationists unwittingly convey the notion that rehabilitation is a kind of endgame, that is, when rehabilitation is over, that is the end of positive change. At least that is what many families and persons with chronic aphasia report they have understood their clinicians to communicate. This is the basis of their frustration and despair when formal rehabilitation ends and aphasia still lingers.

Certainly the structure of health care reimbursement plays a huge role in this misperception. Clinicians must stay attuned to the energy of the disability movement, the shared expertise, and the outburst of activity concerning chronic aphasia, and then pass the word along to clients. They are key players in developing the optimism that permits families and aphasic people to grow and change after rehabilitation ends.

Rehabilitation is but the first important step on the long road to living successfully after stroke. It is critical to communicate that message to the people with whom we work. Rehabilitation is not the final step in recovery, it is just the first step in where recovery action is. It is not magic. Clinicians who work in rehabilitation settings must convey the message that life indeed goes on after rehabilitation, and in most cases, life can continue to get better, particularly if attention is paid to aphasia in its chronic stages. When clients and families are encouraged not to expect magic as a feature of the rehabilitation process, they are far less likely to be disappointed and discouraged.

### Solving the Rehabilitation Mystery: Learning the Rehabilitation Ropes

Just as rehabilitation is not magic, it should not be a mystery either. Box 6–6 lists family members' needs at the outset of speech-language treatment, that is, when clients enter rehabilitation.

At this point, families and aphasic clients are still new not only to aphasia but also to the routines and goals of rehabilitation. Audrey's clinical experience indicates that the majority of people do not fully understand what the therapy process entails, and perhaps most new clinicians do not, either. Accordingly, clinicians need to

---

**Box 6–6. Family Member-Suggested Information Needs at Onset of Speech-Language Treatment**

- What is the purpose of testing?
- What is the purpose of treatment?
- Can we watch or participate in therapy?
- How can we improve interactions?
- How can we help?
- Of what other things should we be aware?
- Is there someone we can talk to who has gone through this?

(From Avent et al., 2005.)

explain to families why tests are given, and also what the treatment is expected to accomplish.[5] Communication counselors need to view families and aphasic persons as fellow experts who can be extremely informative during treatment. Shadden (2005) points out that counselors need to know something about "the relational dynamics in families, going well beyond questions such as, 'How does he communicate at home?'" Issues such as this all require counseling skills.

Families need instruction in supported communication (Kagan, 1998) during formal rehabilitation. In my experience, this typically is postponed until aphasia has become chronic—and thus after the affected person's sense of self has been damaged (although it could have been protected by this approach) (Holland & Beeson, 1993). Is there peer support for families undergoing rehabilitation, or will it have to wait until after rehabilitation? How do we help families to find information and peer support? These are counseling tasks as well.

Rehabilitation is better and easier to tolerate when the participants clearly understand it and consider themselves part of the process. The list of family needs in Box 6–6 also underscores families' concerns about what they should to be doing in the baffling new situation called rehabilitation. For aphasic persons in a rehabilitation center, the daily routine entails living in rooms with strangers; following a relatively rigid schedule; wearing clothes that are possibly unacceptable in one's everyday sartorial world; sitting across a table from a clinician likely to be the age of one's child (or grandchild); and following directions to participate in drills and school-like tasks; not being able to lie down and rest when tired; and eating from a limited menu. The rehabilitation milieu can certainly be managed more comfortably if its participants understand its rules, its goals, and its processes. (Language disorders probably complicate every aspect of this understanding.)

Furthermore, family members and aphasic persons themselves know very little about aphasia before it happens to them, even if Uncle Ted had a stroke some years ago and had trouble talking. One reason for this lack of knowledge is that aphasia is scarcely

---

[5]In many instances, the explanations we give to others also can clarify our own understanding of why we do what we do.

a household word (neither are cognitive-communication problem, dysphagia, apraxia of speech, or dysarthria, for that matter). Furthermore, the sense of crisis may be overwhelming, and the cause of the aphasia, unlike a natural disaster or even a well-publicized illness with glamorous spokespersons such as breast cancer, hardly makes it exotic. Finally, because of aphasia's variability, Uncle Ted's problems probably will not be particularly relevant.[6]

Particularly if they buy into "rehabilitation magic" and are bewildered by "rehabilitation mystery," both aphasic persons and their family members may very well feel uninformed and confused. In such instances, clinical intervention is not likely to be very meaningful, follow-through is negligible, and effectiveness is minimized. Such situations constitute fertile ground for "counseling moments" to occur, and such encounters should be encouraged. If therapy just "happens," without both family and patient buy-in, clinical effectiveness is minimized. Consider the following comment from the spouse of an aphasic man: "As a regular observer and frequent participant in his SLP sessions I felt the sessions were successful primarily in identifying what he could not do" (Quann, 2002, p. 72).

The man, John Quann, was at a rehabilitation center after a stroke. His spouse, Eileen Quann, bright and curious and a true "John Quann expert," was knowledgeable about his former career at NASA before retirement. After observing a session in which he failed utterly at a sequencing task, she chose to recast it to reflect his interests, and the next day he successfully carried out the task with Eileen. Her sequencing task for John was far more demanding than the clinician's original one: She asked him to sequence the planets in order of their distance from the sun. (John also graciously pointed out that she had forgotten to include the now-demoted planet Pluto.) Family as expert cannot be discounted. We need to welcome their involvement. Communication counselors should ask families to partner in the specification and content of materials so that treatment tasks become personally relevant. This

---

[6]Avent and colleagues' questions could well be the comprehensive examination questions for graduate students working on a master's degree in communication disorders. In fact, two of these researchers, Avent and Glista, ask their students to answer them—all of them—as an exercise (J. Avent & S. Glista, personal communication, 2006). Audrey has done this and found that it is not an easy task.

inclusive approach will honor family members' expertise while simultaneously increasing their understanding of aphasia.

We have already mentioned Diane Ackerman and her role in reestablishing her husband's quality of life. The approach she describes was begun well after his return home, and only after a long period of formal therapy. We can only wonder if the healing she describes could have happened earlier if the "experts" had sought her advice, and made her a part of their team.

Consideration of some likely "counseling moments" is appropriate here. Some possibilities are included in Boxes 6–7 and 6–8. Box 6–7 focuses on concerns of persons who experience the disorders; Box 6–8, on concerns of families. Such "counseling moments," of course, can arise at any time, but most are particularly relevant for the rehabilitation center setting and for clinical intervention that may follow it.

## After the Rehabilitation Center

Box 6–9 completes Avent and colleagues' list of perceived needs after leaving the rehabilitation center, or perhaps when health insurance benefits run out. Note that the tenor of the questions has changed. Now they focus on getting on with life. An important source of useful answers to this list of questions and many additional ones is *The Aphasia Handbook*, a handbook developed at Connect, the pioneering British center for persons with chronic aphasia and their families. Its American version is available through the National Aphasia Association (Sarno & Peters, 2004). Communication counselors are urged to make it available to their clients and families as soon as possible upon return to home or to other housing.

There has been an explosion of DVDs, videotapes, and YouTube offerings on living with aphasia, and many of them available at the time of this writing (but certainly not all) are listed at the end of this chapter. We have found such a list to be useful (and it is great fun to surf for them every few months or so), particularly when the focus is on the reestablishment, or perhaps reconstruction, of one's life in familiar surroundings once again. One advantage of these videos and DVDs is that virtually all of them feature people with aphasia who are going about the business of getting on with life.

**Box 6–7. "Counseling Moments" with Individual Clients Expected to Improve/Stabilize**

The following comments from adult clients with communication disorders define clinical scenarios that result in specific "counseling moments." For each scenario, decide whether the "counseling moment," together with the requisite response, is something that is within your scope of practice. If you feel it is not, then answer from that perspective. If you decide it is within your scope of practice, answer from that perspective. (These example "moments" have some overlap with those for parents and children, as listed in Chapters 4 and 5; some also are repeated in Box 6–8, for family/partner issues.)

"Funny thing . . . I got kinda lost in our own house yesterday."

"I know . . . what's wrong, but my kids—no way."

"I could live with this laryngectomy if I was sure I wouldn't get cancer again."

"No f-f-f-food. Why? Why?"

"Our friends don't call me or come over any more."

"I know why . . . Speech . . . here (points around room) . . . good. You listen. Home, family, no!

Family: 'Do your homework!' but just listen? Forget it"

But the bundles on the tarrapoi, say buddy . . . wagerstola."
"What's wrong with me? I know it—can't say it."

"It's all my fault. I messed up. Me! My fault!"

"I hate these hearing aids! Number one, I don't think I need them. If people spoke up, all would be fine. Number two, there is so much noise when I *do* wear them. Number three, they make me look old and unattractive!"

"Why does everyone act like there's something wrong with me? I know I have this trouble walking (points to left leg), but I don't even know why I come to see you! I'm just fine with my thinking."

**Box 6–8. "Counseling Moments" with Families and Partners of Persons Expected to Improve/Stabilize**

The following comments from partners and families define clinical scenarios that result in "counseling moments" specific for this counseling clientele. Perform the same exercises as outlined for Box 6–7.

"If I could just get my mother to come to spouse group, I think a lot of things would fall into place."

"I keep trying to tell my dad that he's got to stop working in the garden when it's so hot. I worry about him all the time."

"Jake got really angry at me last night. I just couldn't figure out what he wanted."

"I think I understand about aphasia, but this seems to be lost on our teenagers."

"Ever since the accident, I keep wondering when the bad dream will be over and Cassie will be her old self again."

"It's all my fault. Stuff like this happens all the time and messes up everything I do."

"I wish I could figure it out. Nothing like this ever happened to me before. I suppose it is just one isolated instance, and I shouldn't worry, right?"

"It makes me feel terrible that I have to lie to him so I can get him back to the nursing home without a scene and a tantrum. The only way I can get him into the car is to tell him we're going shopping or something, and by the time he gets back there, he forgets and it's okay. But I feel like a hypocrite."

"I have no time for me anymore."

The final counseling moment here is somewhat different. What do we do about family members who speak for their communicatively disordered member? Here is a scenario related to that problem:

Clinician (to Brian, the person with aphasia): "Well, Brian, did you have a busy weekend?"

Loretta (Brian's wife): "We sure did. All of the children and grandchildren came over for a barbecue on Saturday, and Sunday we went to the movies after church."

---

**Box 6–9. Family Member Information Needs After Discharge from Speech-Language Treatment**

■ What alternative therapies or activities are available?
■ Whom can we call when we have questions?
■ What else can help at home?
■ Where can we get travel information?
■ Is job training available?
■ What support services are available?
■ What resources are available for long-range planning?

(From Avent et al., 2005.)

---

Although these people do not downplay the problems of living with aphasia, they are eager to encourage others to follow their example, and they are frequently exuberant about sharing their messages of hope with others. We believe that they have potential for truly inspiring others, and that they are especially effective for persons with aphasia and their families as they return to what is the more normal existence of life at home. In addition to the YouTube offerings, tapes, and DVDs, rehab clinicians should match a few of their favorites to the problems a specific client will face upon discharge (i.e., people who remain mostly nonverbal, younger people with aphasia, etc.)

### Living Well with Disability

Without doubt, aphasic people can continue to regain many communication skills after formal rehabilitation. But then the emphasis for communication counseling changes. The challenge for people with aphasia, or other disorders characterized by the likelihood of clinical improvement, is to begin the task of learning to adapt, and to live with disability. In her novel *Birds of a Feather*, Jacqueline Winspear (2004, p. 221) gets it just about right. Her heroine, Maisie Dobbs, is talking to Dr. Dene, an expert in rehabilitation of soldiers wounded in the First World War:

> MAISIE: Tell me, Dr. Dene, if you were to name one thing that made the difference between those who get well and quickly and those who don't, what would it be?
>
> DR. DENE: Well, if I were to name one thing it would be acceptance.
>
> MAISIE: Acceptance? But doesn't that stop the injured or wounded from trying to get better?
>
> DR. DENE: In my opinion, acceptance has to come first. Some people don't accept what has happened. They are stuck at the point of the event that caused the injury.

Maisie then asks Dr. Dene how people "get over" being stuck.

> DR. DENE: I would say it is threefold. One is accepting what has happened. Three is having a picture, an idea of what they will do, when they are better, or improved. Then in the middle, is a path to follow.

Helping to set the "path to follow" is the initial counseling task after rehabilitation. As families and individuals begin to live into their futures, a distinctive counseling role is to help guide acceptance and acknowledgment in ways that permit and encourage living successfully and fully, despite communication problems. The goal is to fit the disability in, not get over it.

Kagan and Simmons-Mackie (2007) describe what they call "beginning with the end."

> We believe what they mean is for people with aphasia and their families, as well as their clinicians and counselors, to

begin the long recovery process by jointly determining where one can expect to be, say, a year or so from now. From our perspective, this is a process not to be determined until formal rehabilitation has worked its wonders, or lack thereof, and when acceptance as Dr. Dene defines it has set in. "The end" for Dr. Dene is what they will do when they are better or improved—and so too for aphasia. Fictional Dr. Dene's "path" is the route of Simmons-Mackie and Kagan as well. It begins at the end of rehab, and fills in the next year, or two, or possibly even more.

The following poem addresses this goal well:

"The Cure"

We think we get over things. We don't get over things

Or say, we get over the measles but not a broken heart. We need to make that distinction.

The things that become a part of our experience never become less a part of our experience.

How can I say it?

The way to "get over" a life is to die. Short of that, you move with it.

Let the pain be pain, not in the hope that it will vanish

But in the faith that it will fit in.

Find its place in the shape of things

And be then not any less pain but true to form. Because anything natural has an inherent shape And it will flow towards it.

And a life is as natural as a leaf. That's what we're looking for.

Not the end of a thing, but the shape of it. Wisdom is seeing the shape of your life

Without obliterating (getting over) a single instant of it.

—Albert Huffstickler (1989)

Communication counselors also are urged to read Pound's article "Dare to Be Different: The Person and the Practice" (2004). Pound writes from her dual perspectives as an SLP and as a person who has learned to live with chronic pain. Box 6–10 describes her particularly well-informed beliefs about appropriate clinician behavior.

Although the course of change is toward improvement, it is both unpredictable and slow. Accordingly, both affected persons and their families should continue to engage in positive, disciplined behaviors designed to promote change and growth, for virtually the rest of their lives. For communicatively disordered persons, this can mean continuing to participate in therapy, or for many aphasic persons, helping others by participating in research projects designed to further current understanding of language disorders. Volunteering to be of service to others often is a meaningful activity as well. Commitment to full living may mean getting healthier, getting closer to one's children and grandchildren, taking more time to relax in a mindful way, learning things one never had time for before, and so forth. The following examples describe ways that two different aphasic persons chose to get on with life:

---

**Box 6–10. How to Act as a Clinician Counselor**

- Act as a reference point.
- Act as a guide.
- Act as an advocate.
- Act as an interpreter.
- Help enable the aphasic client to feel like a person instead of a patient.
- Balance your professional expertise and confidence with listening and exploring "therapist naiveté" (issues of which you have little or no knowledge).
- Train other rehabilitation team members to be skilled conversation partners.

---

(Modified from Pound, 2004.)

Roger Ross,[7] who had very significant aphasia, demonstrated the benefit of positive disciplined behavior. Every morning of his life after his stroke, he read for an hour, moving from simple aphasia-friendly text early on to a point years down the road when he could once again manage his favorite fiction writers, as well as the political science works and current affairs books that had always been his love. Roger read much more slowly than before his stroke, a fact of his aphasia that he acknowledged and accepted. His efforts illustrate growth and change in chronic communication problems. Such growth involves a willingness to work to change what makes personal sense to change and to be curious about how change occurs. It also involves willingness to make peace gracefully with what cannot be changed. Ross, for example, could have easily worked on his writing, as writing was his clear communicative strength. He chose not to do so, arguing that it took time away from what was more important to him: talking better and reading more efficiently.

LC lived fully, as well. But he did it differently—he just got back to the exuberant life he had lived before his stroke. LC also had very significant aphasia. When he realized that his golf game had barely been touched by his stroke, he returned to playing at least once a week. A particular joy for him was playing with strangers at a public course and managing not to reveal his language problem: "Those old guys . . . how about that? They didn't . . . Me? Not talkin' much." He also had at least one weekly lunch with friends. He went to plays and movies and took long trips in his car. He delivered Meals on Wheels, and he volunteered as a guide at a hospital. When I asked him how could provide directions around the hospital when his speech was so littered with paraphasias and difficult to understand, he smiled: "I don't talkin'. Nothing wrong in my wheat, seat, feet—I take 'em there."

---

[7]Roger Ross is his real name—he forbade the use of initials or pseudonyms, saying he was who he was and working to improve the lot of persons with aphasia. Roger Ross's inspirational videotape for aphasic persons is available through the University of Arizona Department of Speech, Language, and Hearing Sciences.

Other aphasic people and their families have described this graceful making of peace in various ways:

"It is a good retirement—just not quite the one we planned."

—Spouse of an aphasic woman, whose stroke occurred immediately following their very carefully planned retirement

"I would say we are contented and lead a good life. But it is a different contentment and a different life."

—Spouse of an aphasic man

"My own journey to "stroke-land" was different from any journey I'd taken before, but it was worth all the effort because I learned to laugh at myself and to trust myself. Before the stroke, I wouldn't have been able to see a brain attack as an opportunity for growth, but it gave me the chance to delve deep inside myself and find that I was tougher than I thought possible." (Perez, 2001)

"Aphasia is just our new normal."

—Spouse of an aphasic man

"Aphasia? I don't think about it anymore." (Ross, 2002) (This statement comes, paradoxically, from the videotape Ross made to inspire other persons with aphasia.)

Doing what needs to be done and what feels right for each individual—whether it is continuing to participate in aphasia groups, getting back to an exercise routine, taking a course in gardening, or moving on and letting go—takes time. It cannot be rushed. Many people with aphasia report that it took longer than a year before things started to seem bright again (see Holland, 2006, for more detailed discussion.)

A word of caution: Clinicians often have biases about what ought to happen or how it should happen. Biases are pernicious and often hard to recognize, but such "shoulds and oughts" are unacceptable in clinical contexts. A client with chronic aphasia who says "enough!" (or perhaps "more!") is to be respected and supported, even when we think we would make a different decision.

## Groups and Group Counseling

Group intervention is a major instrument in the clinician's counseling toolbox for chronic phases of disorders characterized by clinical improvement or stabilization. Moreover, it is no surprise that not only has group treatment post-rehab grown in a time of decreased funding for individual treatment, and as it has, clinicians have increasingly discovered their value in addressing long-term psychosocial needs. Not only is group treatment increasing, but so is comprehensive, and often intensive, group treatment as exemplified by the growing numbers of aphasia centers nationwide (see Simmons-Mackie, 2011, for a glimpse into this movement.) These safe havens provide group experiences for a few hours a day, most of them for 2 or 3 days per week, and most have complex psychosocial agendas. Group treatment in general is the subject of very useful books by Elman (revised edition, 2007) and Pound, Parr, Lindsey, and Woolf (2000). Both books provide many ideas about activities for groups, as well as how they should be organized and conducted. In the context of counseling, groups offer unique opportunities for individuals and their families to learn from each other and for people to come together in the powerful process of socializing once again.

The goals of groups are much more dependent on clinicians' counseling skills than on their more straightforward language intervention skills. Nevertheless, groups also serve as convenient practice sites for the activities that may be learned in individual sessions. They are also appropriate places for exploring and undertaking some positive psychology exercises, in some cases slightly modified for use by persons with communication disabilities. Some adaptations for use with groups (or with individual clients) are presented later in the chapter, and in Chapter 8 as well. Group work frequently is the catalyst for coming to grips with how life may be changed by the physical, behavioral, and communicative consequences of the disorder. For families, learning to be a part of society again is also foremost, and the same counseling issues and approaches also are appropriate; thus, both groups pose similar challenges for communication counselors.

## Group Leadership Skills

Being a good listener is one of the most important group leadership skills. In the group context, this involves leaving time and space for mulling over what has been said. It also means respecting the fact that the answers may actually lie with the questioner and not in the quick response of the listener. Group silence may be construed as even more oppressive than one-on-one silence, so that the session leader may find it even harder than usual to count to five or so before responding. Leading an aphasia group in the process of developing coherence is particularly difficult. If you can manage to keep quiet long enough, you will soon learn that often someone else in a group situation (aphasia group or otherwise) will say what you were thinking. It helps to remember this while waiting out group silence, or while attempting to facilitate talk among group members.

Self-discipline is a related skill. Because clinicians are so-called normal speakers, they need to be wary of dominating the group interaction, or of attempting to direct it to ensure that all goes well. Self-control, sensitivity, and tact all are involved in making it possible for all group members to have floor time, and opportunities to participate to their own level of satisfaction. The central issue for counselors is being able to relinquish control comfortably. Although Roger Ross ran at least three highly successful groups entirely on his own, he refused to allow clinicians to help him with those groups or even to attend them. Clinicians tend to "take over" and "spoil it," he said (R. Ross, personal communication, discussed in Holland, 2007).

In facilitating aphasia groups, a special responsibility that relies on counseling skills is acting as a "communication broker." It is almost an art to interpret one aphasic group member's somewhat unintelligible communication to other group members who also have aphasia. Clinicians must be prepared to make mistakes while brokering and learn to laugh at them, confident in the knowledge that laughter is an extremely important part of successful clinical intervention.[8]

As mentioned earlier in relation to rehabilitation centers, supported communication is another technical skill essential to successful communication counseling. Teaching its concepts to family members, however, is equally a clinical skill, a counseling issue, and an art. Box 6–11 contains some of the principles of supported communication, as outlined by Kagan (1998 and as expanded on in Simmons-Mackie, King and Beukelman (2013).

---

### Box 6–11. Principles of Supported Communication

*To facilitate comprehension:*

Supplement speech with pictures, objects, and written words or phrases.

Use natural gestures and drawings to augment speech.

Modify speech when appropriate, by slowing down, emphasizing key words, pausing at natural places.

Allow extra time for processing.

Signal speaker change with gaze or natural gesture.

Signal topic change through use of total communication.

Confirm client's understanding.

*To facilitate speaking:*

Encourage total communication; accept any modality used.

Provide relevant pictures, objects, and/or writing for client to use.

Allow extra time for speaking

Model use of total communication strategies.

Facilitate sharing floor time.

Facilitate topic change when conversation lags.

Resist "speaking for" another to the extent it is possible to do so.

---

(Modified from Kagan & Gailey, 1993.)

---

[8]For a thorough discussion of this and other useful notions, see Simmons-Mackie (2004).

Although it is clearly possible to train people in these skills one on one, teaching and practicing them in group settings is particularly effective. More examples can be shared, and for family members, learning these precepts also involves learning more about aphasia and its effects on others' lives. A useful supplement, not only for aphasic families but also for other health care professionals, is the set of guidelines provided by Holland and Halper (1996). Supported communication taught in partner group settings provides an excellent opportunity to facilitate peer role models and shared experiences as well. Although supported communication principles have been developed with aphasic persons in mind, they are applicable across the range of communication disorders associated with likelihood of improvement (with appropriate modification) as well. Elman and Hoover (2013) provide an excellent "how-to" resource.

An additional benefit of supported communication is that it can help adults with communication disorders to develop behaviors that help to put their nonimpaired conversation partner at ease, thereby enhancing communication interaction. These skills are particularly useful for encounters with strangers or occasional interactants. Like supported communication itself, group therapy seems an ideal setting for learning them. Box 6–12 provides some suggestions for ways in which aphasic persons may help conversation partners, with the goal of improving interpersonal interaction.

## Individual Counseling

Communication counselors can have an equally viable role in one-on-one work with persons with communication disabilities. Each of the issues presented for group work can have a starring role in individual therapy as well, including the importance of sharing floor time, and attempting to achieve interactional parity.

One particularly pertinent issue, delicate and difficult to frame, stands out in individual work with adults. The concepts of shared expertise and aiding clients to develop resilience, identity, and self-efficacy seem at odds with traditional SLP-A concepts of feedback and external reinforcement. Arguably important in work with

---

**Box 6–12. For the Poststroke Client:
Helping Others to Help You**

1. Carry a card that explains your problem and what helps you to communicate better. For example:

   My name is Lester Breivold. I had a stroke and can't talk very well. Please be patient with me. I do much better when the other person is patient. I have a pen and notepad, and I may ask you to write a few words to help me sometimes.

2. For clients who are able to learn such a message, it should be spoken as well. For example:

   I am Lester Breivold. I had a stroke. Speaking is difficult. Please be patient with me. I'll help you if I get stuck.

3. Learn what works to facilitate interactions. Ask for the help you need. For example:

   ■ Ask for repeats.
   ■ Ask partner to slow down.
   ■ Ask for the word to be written.
   ■ Ask interactant to look at you.

4. Put the interactant at ease with body language, smiles, and other indicators of good will.

---

children,[9] the use of the judgmental "Good" in its many instantiations, or the dismissive "Not quite—let's try again" in its various forms, can be toxic in work with adults. Judgmental comments about adult clients' performance of clinical tasks probably undermine rapport and mutual respect.

Consider the effect (and the psychological cost) of telling Mr. E, a previously successful and articulate trial lawyer, that his attempt to say the word cat (or even misdemeanor) was "terrific." He knows it was not "terrific"—in fact, he is painfully aware that

---

[9]See Chapter 5 regarding its questionable use with children.

the word he produced was barely recognizable. For this client, pointing out what was wrong with his attempt may be less damaging because it is honest feedback concerning his everyday speech. Wording and content of feedback should be carefully considered for each situation. Box 6–13 presents some alternatives that reflect mutual expertise, are consistent with active positive responding, and do not damage identity.

## Some Positive Interventions for Counseling After Stroke

This section presents four activities from the positive psychology interventions described in Chapter 2 that have been adapted for use with stroke and spouse groups. Chapter 8 provides some coherent models for counseling workshops that are designed to build optimism and resilience in a systematic way, and exercises like these appear there, too. Most of them can be adapted to use with children as well.

### Identifying and Using Signature Strengths

Taking the VIA survey (described in Chapter 2 and available at http://www.authentichappiness.org) is beyond the language skills of many persons who have communication problems after stroke;

---

**Box 6–13. Some Alternatives to
"Good Talking, Mr. Jones"**

- "I'm thinking that sounds a lot better—what do you think?
- "Great, I think you got it. Did you, for real?
- "If you're okay with that, so am I. Do you think the family will understand?"
- "You know what? I don't think your kids will get that."
- "Sometimes trying again helps—let's see if it helps you here!"
- "Let's check to see if your message got through."

however, it is relatively easy to adapt the principles of the VIA for use as the basis for a group discussion, as follows:

After the importance of using character strengths is introduced, each group participant is given a set of color-coded cards with one of the 24 character strengths written on each (e.g., strengths of wisdom and knowledge on green cards, strengths of transcendence on purple, and so on). All cards should be in the same order (not determined by color code) to facilitate use by readers and non-readers both. The group leader reads each card aloud and asks the participants to decide if the strength is "like me," "not like me," or "not sure," and then to place the cards on one of three stacks labeled YES, NO, and ??, respectively. When all 24 cards have been considered, participants go through their YES cards again, looking for the five that are most like them. These become the basis for exploring character strengths and virtues, what the color coding means, and so forth. Some possible illustrative questions follow:

- Are your five top cards all the same color? What does it mean?
- What does it mean if they are not?
- Was it easy to find cards that describe you?
- Did you have more than five cards?
- Which category makes the biggest of your stacks? (like me, not like me, not sure)
- From your "like me" stack, pick the one that describes you best. How did that strength help you most when you had a stroke?

This activity can be used with family groups as well, without the prompts by the group leader, and in a less tightly constrained form. For both groups, the relevant follow-up activity is to use one of the top five strengths during the next week, making the experience the basis for the next week's discussion.

## A Good Thing Happened

"A Good Thing Happened" is an adaptation of the "Three Good Things" exercise (which can be used in its original form with partners and families). The concept embodied in this exercise is useful as a focus for group interaction or as an individual conversation topic. The clinician provides a personal example first and then asks each participant to tell of one good thing that happened during the week, using principles of supported communication to evoke the incidents, where necessary. All are written down for participants to study. Then the clinician uses his or her own example as the stimulus for the question "What did I do to bring it about?" Again, answers are supported and written. The only wrong answer is "I didn't do anything—it just happened." That is the answer that everyone gets to challenge. For example:

CLIENT: Real good chocolate cone yesterday.

CLINICIAN: How did you bring that about?

CLIENT: Dunno . . . happened.

CLINICIAN: Not true! Did you decide when you saw the Häagen-Dazs store? Did you ask Mabel to get it? What?

The point of this exercise is to provide practice in taking responsibility not only for the bad things that happen in life but for the good ones as well. This is not always easy and in itself constitutes an excellent discussion topic.

### Positive Consequences of Stroke

Look back at Box 6–3. It contains an unplanned moment of high positivity, and clinicians must always be on the lookout for them; however, it is also possible to engineer such moments. This next exercise probably works best with people who have been living with their impairments for some time. It also may serve as a useful introduction for a new member of a group, particularly if the older members have practiced it before, and take the lead in sharing their answers with the new member. It is equally appropriate for families. The stimulus topic can be presented as follows:

"We spend a lot of time thinking about the problems that result from stroke. It's important to talk about them, but it is also a good idea to see if anything at all good came out of the stroke."

The clinician can provide examples such as the one from Box 6–3, but much simpler examples are acceptable as well.[10]

### Gratitude Visit

Families and affected persons are encouraged to work together on planning and carrying out a gratitude visit, as outlined in Chapter 2. In addition, however, an appropriate form of the poststroke gratitude visit is to direct the visit to someone who has been particularly helpful since the stroke, that is, someone who has made the adaptation process easier.

### Stroke and Successful Living

This has been just a brief smattering of ideas, and more are presented in Chapter 8, along with exercises for increasing resilience and optimism. One underlying theme of such interventions is that attempting a working balance of all aspects of PERMA is a privilege to be enjoyed by everyone, including persons whose abilities have been compromised by an unexpected event. The exercises should serve as a reminder that the path to flourishing, even for the disabled, is really a two-way path. It is not just receiving gifts, cards, and letters from friends, but also giving or sending them; not just getting one's communication supported by others, but also helping others to be at ease in the presence of a communication disorder; not just learning to laugh again, but perhaps also learning to make others laugh. Such considerations are part of the larger picture of successful living, with or without disability.

Regardless of its focus on stroke, almost all of the concepts, principles, and exercises presented here can be applied in counseling and coaching for the other disorders with progression toward improvement/stabilization. Translation for application to those other disorders of course involves careful consideration of causes, specific facts of the disorders, and attributes of their treatment, but the principles and the issues remain largely the same: the concepts of building resilience and optimism, focusing on strength, telling

---

[10]One client said, "My daughter now calls us every weekend." Audrey's own favorite is from an inspirationally positive aphasic man: "It got me a 'Handicapped' sticker for my car."

stories, and sharing expertise apply to the gamut from presbycusis to TBI. For example, the program in learning to live successfully with hearing loss described by Marrone and Harris (2012) shares strikingly similar principles and techniques to those presented here.

## References

Ackerman, D. (2011). *One hundred names for love: A memoir.* New York, NY: W. W. Norton.

Avent, J., Glista, S., Wallace, S., Jackson, J., Nishioka, J., & Yip, W. (2005). Family information needs about aphasia. *Aphasiology, 19*, 365–375.

Berger, P., & Mensch, S. (1999). *How to conquer the world with one hand and an attitude.* Merrifield, VA: Positive Power.

Douglas, K. (2003). *My stroke of luck.* New York, NY: Macmillan.

Dow, D. (2013). *Brain attack: My journey of recovery from stroke and aphasia.* Henderson NV: Speechless Publishing.

Elman, R. (Ed.). (2007). *Group treatment of neurogenic communication disorders: The expert clinician's approach* (Rev. ed.). San Diego, CA: Plural.

Elman, R., & Hoover, E. (2013). Integrating communication support into aphasia group treatment. In N. Simmons-Mackie, J. King, & D. Beukelman (Eds.), *Supporting communication for adults with acute and chronic aphasia.* Baltimore, MD: Paul H. Brookes.

Godecke, E., Hird, K., Lalor, E., Rai, T., & Phillips, M. (2012). Very early post stroke aphasia therapy: A pilot randomized controlled efficacy trial. *International Journal of Stroke, 7*, 635–644.

Helm-Estabrooks, N. (2002). Cognition in aphasia: A discussion and a study. *Journal of Communication Disorders, 35*, 171–186.

Hinckley, J. (2006). Finding messages in bottles: Living successfully with stroke and aphasia. *Topics in Stroke Rehabilitation, 13*, 25–35.

Holland, A. (2006). Living successfully with aphasia: Three variations on a theme. *Topics in Stroke Rehabilitation, 13*, 44–51.

Holland, A. (2007). The power of aphasia groups: Celebrating Roger Ross. In Elman, R. (Ed.). *Group treatment of neurogenic communication disorders: The expert clinician's approach* (rev. ed.). San Diego, CA: Plural.

Holland, A., & Beeson, P. (1993). Finding oneself following stroke. A reply to Brumfitt's "Losing one's sense of self following stroke." *Aphasiology, 7*, 581–583.

Holland, A., & Fridriksson, J. (2001). Management for aphasia in the acute phases post stroke. *American Journal of Speech-Language Pathology, 10*(1), 19–28.

Holland, A., & Halper, A. (1996). Communicating with individuals who are aphasic. *Topics in Aphasia Rehabilitation, 2,* 37–34.

Holland, A., & Ramage, A. (2004). Learning from Roger Ross: A clinical journey. In J. F. Duchan & S. Byng (Eds.), *Challenging aphasia therapies.* New York, NY: Psychology Press.

Huffstickler, A. (1989). The cure. In A. Huffsickler & C. Bogen (Eds.), *Walking wounded.* Austin, TX: Backyard Press.

Kagan, A. (1998). Supported conversation for adult with aphasia: Methods and resources for training conversational partners. *Aphasiology, 12,* 816–830.

Kagan, A., & Gailey, G. (1993). Functional is not enough. Training conversation partners for aphasic adults. In A. Holland & M. Forbes (Eds.), *Aphasia treatment: World perspectives* (pp. 199–225). San Diego, CA: Singular.

Kagan, A., & Simmons-Mackie, N. (2007). Beginning with the end: Outcome-driven assessment and treatment with life participation in mind. *Topics in Language Disorders, 27,* 309–317.

Kagan A., Simmons-Mackie N., Rowland A., Huijbregts M., Shumway E., McEwen S., . . . Sharp, S. (2007) Counting what counts: A framework for capturing real-life outcomes of aphasia intervention. *Aphasiology, 22,* 258–280.

Marrone, N., & Harris, F. P. (2012). A multifaceted living well approach to the management of hearing loss with adults and their frequent communication partners. *Perspectives on Aural Rehabilitation and Its Instrumentation, 19,* 5–14.

Mayer, T. (2000). *One handed in a two-handed world* (2nd ed.). Boston, MA: Prince-Gallison Press.

McCrum, R. (1999). *My year off: Recovering life after a stroke.* New York, NY: Broadway Books.

National Institute of Mental Health. (2006). *Depression and stroke fact sheet.* Retrieved from http://www.nimh.nih.gov

Peach, R. (2001). Further thoughts regarding management of acute aphasia following stroke. *American Journal of Speech Language Pathology, 10,* 29–36.

Perez, P. (2001). *Brain attack: Danger, chaos, opportunity, empowerment.* Johnson, VT: Cutting Edge Press.

Pound, C. (2004). Dare to be different: The person and the practice. In J. F. Duchan & S. Byng (Eds.), *Challenging aphasia therapies.* New York, NY: Psychology Press.

Pound, C., Parr, S., Lindsay, J., & Woolf, C. (2000). *Beyond aphasia: Therapies for living with communication disability.* Bicester, UK: Winslow.

Quann, E. (2002). *By his side: Life and love after stroke.* Highland, MD: Fastrack.

Reivich, K., & Shatté, A. (2002). *The resilience factor: Seven essential skills for overcoming life's inevitable obstacles.* New York, NY: Broadway Books.

Robey, R. (1998). A meta-analysis of clinical outcomes in the treatment of aphasia. *Journal of Speech Language and Hearing Research, 41,* 172–187.

Sarno, M. T., & Peters, J. (2004). *The aphasia handbook* (USA ed.). Retrieved from http://www.aphasia.org

Shadden, B. (2005). Aphasia as identity theft: Theory and practice. *Aphasiology, 19,* 211–224.

Simmons-Mackie, N. (2004). Just kidding: Humor and therapy for aphasia. In J. F. Duchan & S. Byng (Eds.), *Challenging aphasia therapies.* New York, NY: Psychology Press.

Simmons-Mackie, N. (Ed.). (2011). Aphasia centers: A growing trend in North America. *Seminars in Speech and Language, 32,* 3.

Simmons-Mackie, N., King, J., & Beukelman, D. (2013) *Supporting communication for adults with acute and chronic aphasia.* Baltimore, MD: Paul H. Brookes.

Stroke Connection. American Stroke Association. Retrieved from http://www.strokeassociation.org

Stroke Smart. National Stroke Association. Retrieved from http://www.stroke.org

Wender, D. (1989). Aphasic victim as investigator. *Archives of Neurology, 46,* 91–92.

Winspear, J. (2004). *Birds of a feather.* New York, NY: Penguin Press.

## Selected Videos, Films, and Internet Websites for Aphasic Individuals and Families on Stroke and Its Consequences

Anatomy of a Comeback: The Sean Maloney Story[a]

Adler Aphasia Center: http://www.Adleraphasiacenter.org[a]

Afterwords (National Aphasia Association)

Aphasia: The Movie (Best Short Film 2010)

Aphasia Center of West Texas website—Ann's message about aphasia: http://aphasiawtx.org

---

[a]Available on YouTube™.

Aphasia Hope Foundation: http://www.aphasiahope.org

American Stroke Association, a division of the American Heart Association: http://www.strokeassociation.org

Inside Aphasia (2007). Available through the Callier Center, Dallas TX

McWreath, J. M. (2006). Picturing aphasia. Video tape. Available at: http://www.aphasia.tv

National Aphasia Association: http://www.aphasia.org

National Stroke Association: http://www.stroke.org

Ross, R. (2002). Living successfully with aphasia. Videotape (available from the University of Arizona Department of Speech, Language, and Hearing Sciences, Tucson AZ).

Sean Maloney rowing video[a]

Talk to Me 1 and 2 (Snyder Center for Aphasic Life Enhancement: SCALE) [a]

The David Dow Story[a]

---

[a]Available on YouTube™.

# Chapter 7

# COMMUNICATION COUNSELING WITH ADULT CLIENTS AND THEIR FAMILIES FOR WHOM EXPECTED PROGRESSION IS TOWARD DETERIORATION

## Introduction

Most communication counselors eventually encounter some clients with disorders that are not expected to change for the better and for which the best outcomes are maintaining the current levels of impairment and functioning for as long as possible. Such disorders are collectively referred to here as *disorders of downward progression* (in contrast to the disorders discussed in Chapter 6, which typically show improvement and upward progress). They include Parkinson disease (PD), amyotrophic lateral sclerosis (ALS), Huntington disease (HD), the variants of cerebellar degeneration, supranuclear palsy, and, except for the few reversible ones, the entire range of dementias. These disorders worsen over time despite the best current medical and behavioral practices. They probably reflect a greater challenge to communication counselors than most of the other disorders discussed in this book. Not only is dissolution of speech, language, swallowing, and cognition a concern, but end-of-life issues also appear.

Furthermore, older children potentially have a role in making decisions and sharing responsibilities for issues ranging from finances to housing to end-of-life concerns. This is somewhat true for individuals who have aphasia and the other disorders discussed in Chapter 6, of course, but it is likely to be even more pervasive here. The counseling issues do not necessarily change, but the potential for a variety of differing views increases. Alert communication counselors should attempt to understand the family dynamics that might be at play.

As might be expected, depression is common among people who have these disorders as well as their families. A prevailing myth is that persons with dementia are often spared from depression. This is not so, but the probability of it lessens after a dementing person has experienced major deterioration. For SLPs, the challenge of disorders of downward progression is somewhat mitigated by the fact that we are only infrequently the central counselors. Nevertheless, our counseling role is important and our responsibilities are unique. Box 7–1 presents some "counseling moments" for practice.

The disorders of downward progression also present challenges to the practice of positive psychology and to the development of hope and resilience. Nonetheless, what follows is not a rehearsal of despair, or of merely coping. We suggest a number of ways to make the most out of life, despite the conditions that signal its end.

The chapter begins with a brief discussion of mild cognitive impairment (MCI), a term that has come into vogue for describing a range of memory problems between benign memory loss in aging and very early-onset dementia. MCI is included here,

## Box 7–1. "Counseling Moments" with Families, Affected Persons, and Staff in Extended Care Facilities

The following comments from families, affected persons, and staff define different clinical scenarios in extended care facilities. Decide whether the resulting "counseling moment," along with the response you make to it, is within your scope of practice. If you feel it is not, then craft an appropriate answer.

For families:

"We live a life of isolation since the dementia started to get worse. We have no friends and no social life."

"I keep trying to tell my dad that he's got to stop working in the garden when it's so hot. After all, he has Mom to take care of, and he needs to be healthy. I worry about him all the time."

"It's really getting worse every day. I hardly sleep, I'm losing weight, I have no energy or ambition, and I am wondering if it's worth it to keep on trying. "

"I'm worried about the kids being around him. Is multiple sclerosis contagious?"

"I know I am a worrier, but I have a lot of trouble remembering names, and I get very distracted when there is too much noise. I keep thinking I'm getting Old Timer's Disease."

"I'm not getting any help from his children, and I simply can't manage him at home anymore."

"We've been worrying about Mom ever since Dad died a few years ago. It's only getting worse. She seems so fragile and failing. Her memory is going, and last week, her neighbors called to say she was wandering around, lost. The fact that we live over an hour away is really scary. What do you think we ought to do?"

For persons with the disorders:

"The doctor tells me I have Lou Gehrig's disease. But I really don't understand what that will mean for me. You have been very helpful with my swallowing. Can you send me to a good website so I can get more information?"

"I feel like my mind is dissolving. It's really getting worse every day. I hardly sleep, I am losing weight, I have no energy or ambition. I am wondering if it's worth it to keep on trying." (From a patient with PD)

"I want to die."

"I know I should be practicing those exercises with you today. But I'm down. I have the feeling I brushed my own teeth for the last time this morning." (From a patient with nonbulbar ALS)

"I had a visit from Mama last night. It was so nice to see her." (From an 80-year-old nursing home resident with AD)

"I have problems remembering names, and I sometimes have to look far and wide before I find what I am looking for. My family doesn't notice, but I am wondering if I am getting Alzheimer disease."

For extended care facility staff:

"It sure would be nice if somebody had some ideas about making this place work better."

"I really go nuts when Mrs. Sertnus keeps saying, 'Help me!' She only wants attention, you know."

"If we can't figure out some way to get Mr. Finchley to eat, he's gonna end up with a plug, or dead!"

even though it does not necessarily even count as a "disorder" but is increasingly becoming an area of interest for SLP-As. It presents a challenging counseling issue for us. The chapter then focuses on two quite distinct classes of disorders—one predominantly motor, the other cognitive. We illustrate each class by providing a single example of each. Amyotrophic lateral sclerosis (ALS) serves as our example of motor disorders because it is among the most complex, involving counseling issues concerning its management as well as dealing with end-of-life issues. Dementia is our cognitive example. We define it broadly here, that is, as a spectrum ranging from Alzheimer disease (AD) (probably the most prevalent) to primary progressive aphasia (PPA) (possibly the most clearly relevant for communication counselors). Following the pattern of previous chapters, the salient counseling characteristics of each disorder are discussed first.

## Mild Cognitive Impairment

Mild cognitive impairment (MCI) is a loss of memory, naming impairment, and other cognitive changes that occur both in normal aging and dementing disorders. The determination of MCI is made for individuals who report such problems but also can carry on their normal everyday routines and activities with their usual level of independence. Frequently, even close others may not notice the difficulties with rapid recall of proper names, taking longer to remember where something was put for a few minutes, or forgetting to make a scheduled phone call that might well plague the older person who is fully aware of the existence of the problems. But the devil truly resides in the simple detail that currently there is no way to determine if MCI will develop into a dementia (typically AD or PPA), or will just remain as "senior moments" possibly of increasing frequency. In our experience, a growing number of individuals who are diagnosed as having MCI are being referred to speech, language, and hearing clinics seeking guidance and advice from SLP-As. This is because of our knowledge both of good techniques for improving attention and listening, memory, and word recall skills (gained from our work with individuals who have incurred hearing loss, TBI, aphasia, and to some degree, early dementia and PPA). MCI is mentioned here largely because it has many of the counseling issues accompanying disorders of downward progression. This is not the place to outline specific clinical techniques for this very interesting and important segment of the aging population; however, it *is* a place to remind readers that most of the suggestions for counseling suggested here (particularly for groups) can easily be applied. It is also important for communication counselors to remind people with MCI about the value of using strategies to enhance listening and memory skills, develop exercise routines for mind and body, eat healthy Mediterranean diets, and so forth.

## Amyotrophic Lateral Sclerosis

The motor-neuron disease amyotrophic lateral sclerosis (ALS), or Lou Gehrig's disease as it is popularly known, is progressive and fatal. Both upper and lower motor neurons are ultimately involved, and patients lose the ability voluntarily to move their arms, legs, and the muscles involved in speaking and swallowing. Some recent work also suggests that persons with ALS may experience alterations in cognition as the disease progresses (Rippon et al., 2006). Sensory abilities are not affected, and control of eye muscles appears to be intact in even well-advanced ALS. The preservation of eye movement makes it possible for many persons with ALS to use augmentative systems based on visual tracking long after the disease has progressed significantly.[1] Eye-tracking technology is becoming increasingly more sophisticated, and SLPs should make an effort to keep abreast of new devices that have clinical relevance. Ventilation sometimes is used to enhance breathing, but the usual cause of death in ALS is respiratory failure. Although the projected lifespan after its onset typically is 3 to 5 years, and ALS is most likely to occur in middle age, there are frequent exceptions. For example, the physicist Stephen Hawking, arguably the most famous ALS survivor alive today, was diagnosed in his early twenties and currently is in his seventh decade of life, communicating very effectively with a sophisticated augmentative device and living a full, if wheelchair-bound, life.

The National Institute of Neurological Disorders and Stroke (NINDS) notes on the ALS page of the NINDS website that 90% to

---

[1]Insight into the world of such persons can be developed by reading Jean-Claude Beauby's book, *The Diving Bell and the Butterfly* (1998), written only by use of eye movement and the help of his speech therapist. Beauby's disorder was locked-in syndrome resulting from stroke.

95% of persons with ALS appear to have contracted the disease at random and have no clearly associated risk factors. The remaining 5% to 10% of persons with ALS appear to have inherited it, some from a specific genetic defect, which in the future may provide valuable clues for managing ALS-associated neuronal degeneration and death. Although much current research is attempting to isolate the cause of ALS, to understand the mechanisms involved in its progression, and to provide effective treatment, no clear answers yet exist to help affected persons and their families to deal with these issues.

Furthermore, only one FDA-approved drug for the treatment of ALS—riluzole—currently exists (see the NINDS ALS website). The drug does not cure ALS or reverse existing damage; however, it does appear to reduce (but not eliminate) some further neuron damage by decreasing the release of the neurotransmitter glutamate. Riluzole also appears to retard progression of dysphagia, and to extend the time before a patient requires ventilation. Because of its specific relationship to swallowing, riluzole is of particular significance to communication counselors involved with persons with ALS and their families.

Although ALS can have its earliest manifestations in any muscle group, a substantial number of affected persons have reported initial difficulty in speaking or swallowing or in problems such as choking or drooling. Even early on, persons with this form of ALS often have the telltale sign of tongue fasciculations. This form is known as bulbar ALS, and although dysarthria and dysphagia eventually develop in all persons with ALS, bulbar presentation provides early opportunities and challenges for beneficial and, to some degree, prophylactic intervention by SLPs in both direct treatment and counseling.

The opportunities reside in helping people with ALS and their families to develop proactive management strategies both for dysphagia, which will inevitably worsen, and for dysarthria, which will do the same. Clinicians provide this help by direct suggestions and techniques for "holding the line" as long as possible concerning management of glutition and nutrition, providing direct therapy for its distinctive mixed dysarthria, and helping the affected person and family to choose the most appropriate form of communication augmentation and then providing practice in its use.

The challenges for counseling come about in how we forecast the worsening. Helping the ALS person and his or her significant others to realize and deal with the fact that worsening will occur requires the clinician's counseling skills. Decisions concerning the use of ventilators and tracheotomies become central and therefore are major counseling concerns.

Nevertheless, persons whose ALS is initially bulbar can benefit from early speech-language pathology intervention, just as those with lower or upper extremity problems can benefit from early physical or occupational therapy. SLPs are most likely to encounter clients whose ALS had initial lower extremity expression only later in its course, but because they still can make substantial contributions to managing problems of maintenance and change, the earlier their involvement, the more proactive help SLPs can provide.

The central issues, then, for communication counseling concern the deterioration of function over time in swallowing and speaking, and maintaining quality of life despite it. Part of the problem is how to cope with the erosion of skills, but an equally salient concern is how to make the most of life under such circumstances. These issues are taken up later.

## The Dementias

Management of the spectrum of dementias frequently requires different regimens of medical care, depending on the specific diagnosis; however, the generic label *dementia* (a "wastebasket" term for a number of conditions) is used here. This is primarily because, once the curable and treatable dementias have been eliminated, the basic issues for communication counselors (as opposed to medical personnel) do not appear to require the fine-tuning of more explicit labels. For example, for persons whose dementia is of indeterminate cause and for those who are presumed to have AD, there are few differences in counseling needs.[2]

---

[2]Primary progressive aphasia (PPA) may be an exception, and some of that disorder's unique issues are discussed separately later, when pertinent. Another exception may be multi-infarct dementia. Many of these patients know their families, their own histories, and identity until nearly the end, and this makes a great difference to caregivers.

Most dementias are not in themselves life-threatening. Persons with dementia may live a decade or more after diagnosis and typically die from another condition that may be hastened by the aging process itself, rather than by the dementia. Dementia can be an indirect cause of death, however, as a result of changes in cognitive status. For example, deterioration may increase poor judgment or indifference to safety or nutrition.

A plethora of websites address AD, the most common form of dementia. A few examples, with extensive links to others, are listed at the end of the chapter. These sites describe extensive ongoing scientific research devoted to this problem, as well as a few moving videos and films. Investigators currently are learning much more about the changing neurology and progression of AD. For example, in the rare familial form of early-onset AD, the inheritance pattern has been found to be autosomal dominant, with gene mutations on chromosomes 1, 14, and 21. For later-onset AD (i.e., 60 years of age or older) evidence indicates that persons who inherit one or two copies of the APOE e4allele, as opposed to copies of e2 or e3, on chromosome 19 appear to be at increased risk for AD. Beyond this, however, no clear-cut genetic linkages to AD are known. Other, possibly more environmentally mediated causes of AD, also remain unclear, and pharmaceutical agents, such as galantamine, donepezil, and rivastigmine, have limited effectiveness in slowing early progression in a small number of people. Memantine can offer some limited help at later stages. Even the sources of neuritic plaques and neurofibrillary tangles that are AD's signature pathology remain elusive.[3]

Few other dementias are as well explained as AD. Although progress is constantly being made in understanding, for persons who become demented and for their families, much about the dementias remains as baffling and perplexing as it was nearly two decades ago. SLP-As who work with dementing persons are urged

---

[3]Before leaving the subject of pharmaceutical issues in AD, it seems reasonable to include a cautionary note about medications and aging in general. Regardless of which diseases are the focus, many of the disorders discussed here, as well as those of Chapter 6, bring with them the possibility that individuals who incur them are taking multiple medications, bringing about increased risk of interactive effects on both speech and language and cognition. A good summary for SLP-As is given by Johnson (2013).

to study the comprehensive texts by Bayles and Tomoeda (2007) or Bourgeois and Hickey (2009).

Such matters are at the heart of dementia's counseling issues. Few pharmaceutical or direct behavioral interventions are effective; tremendous family burden often persists for long periods of time; heart-wrenching decisions must be made concerning placement and management. Fortunately, the counseling responsibilities for the dementias are typically spread out over a number of helping professions. It is important, therefore, that health care professionals share the information they provide with other team members. Because deteriorating communication is an ever-present signal of cognitive decline, the role we play is substantial.

Similar to traumatic brain injury (TBI) in this regard, language problems in dementia seldom exist as the central concern; difficulties with memory, executive functioning, or more general cognitive functioning occupy that role. Language, however, is the medium through which persons with dementia express their other cognitive problems and manifest them to their significant others. Also, as with TBI, for clinicians the result is a subtle shift away from interventions directed at improvement of speech, hearing, and language; instead, intervention often focuses on environmental manipulations that support and bolster language and memory. It also includes helping to reduce the effects of these bewildering problems on others in the dementing person's environment. Major differences between TBI and dementia include their typical age of onset and their progression, in the case of TBI toward improvement, and in dementia, toward its downward course. Once again, maintaining function for as long as possible and slowing the rate of decline are goals with persons who have dementia, rather than working to effect lasting improvement, as is the case with TBI.

The issues of ventilators and tracheotomies for persons with advanced motor speech disorders have been mentioned previously, but it seems clear that the counseling issues in dementia are in synchrony with those that arise with use of feeding tubes and other technologies that can possibly extend life. We should be ready to discuss the pros and cons of such interventions with families of dementing persons as well. Again, listening to families, helping them to clarify the issues, and providing valid information to aid in their decision making all require counseling skill. Chapter 9 explores end-of-life issues for SLPs.

## The Concept of Ambiguous Loss

People and families facing disorders of downward progression share what family therapist Pauline Boss calls "ambiguous loss" (1999). Boss defines *ambiguous loss* as loss that remains unclear, indeterminate, and unresolved for some period of time, with a lingering lack of closure and clarity. Ambiguous losses get frozen in time, making it difficult, if not impossible, for grieving and other methods for handling outright loss to be fully exploited. Communication disorders such as those discussed here are not alone as examples of ambiguous loss. Many other medically determined illnesses, such as slow-growing malignant tumors, also can be cited as examples of ambiguous loss.

One of Boss's two major types of ambiguous loss has particular resonance for the disorders of downward progression. Boss characterizes this type of ambiguous loss as that involving "goodbye without leaving" (1999, p. 45).[4] Because of the centrality of disturbed communication and cognitive processes in disorders of downward progression, *goodbye without leaving* is an apt metaphor for people who still are alive but who cannot communicate in their usual style or who have deteriorated in some fundamental ways. Boss's concern is primarily for families in these circumstances, but it seems obvious that people who suffer from ALS or any of the dementias in early stages also feel their own ambiguity in loss of self. They doubtless experience pain when they confront the fact that they are indeed leaving without goodbye. Here, Boss's metaphor, along with her suggestions for handling ambiguous loss, is explored as a counseling focus.

"Goodbye without leaving," in Boss's view, is the most painful form of loss. For persons with disorders such as ALS, the loss becomes more apparent to others as communication progressively fails. The source of the loss in ALS is largely physical. One of the counseling responsibilities with such patients and their families is to provide and then to encourage the use of strategies and devices

---

[4]Boss terms the other type of ambiguous loss "leaving without goodbye." Such losses occur with the disappearance of persons with whom it was not possible to share farewells, such as birth mothers of adopted persons or soldiers who are missing in action.

to augment dwindling skills or to serve as alternative forms of communication, that is, to prevent "goodbye without leaving" for as long as possible. Counselors can help families in strategy development, as in the following example:

> Gideon, a retired man with progressive dementia, has for some time consistently begun his day with a walk to his favorite neighborhood café. He is well known there by both other neighborhood denizens and the café staff, and he always orders the same thing. As his dementia develops, Phoebe, his wife, has become increasingly nervous about this routine and seeks to curtail it. Phoebe is concerned primarily about Gideon's safety, but also about embarrassment for both of them.
>
> A short-term solution involves creative problem solving. For example, perhaps a visit to the café staff, for Phoebe to explain Gideon's new problems and provide guidelines concerning how to handle them, may be of benefit. When Gideon leaves the house, it may be worthwhile to follow him a couple of times to assure Phoebe that he is capable of making the trip alone. Concerning his time at the café, a helpful intervention may be to explain his condition to a few of his café buddies and give them a few suggestions for including him in their conversation.

This approach also is appropriate for persons with PPA, for whom a similar implementation has been well described and documented (Rogers, King, & Alarcon, 2000).

## As Loss Grows More Apparent

Once motor or cognitive difficulties substantially worsen, clinicians face a counseling dilemma related to shared expertise. Is it our responsibility to encourage communication once it becomes exceedingly laborious or, in the case of dementia, when communication becomes manifestly uninteresting to the communicator? Our profession recognizes implicitly that communication, maintained as long as possible, postpones "leaving" in the sense described by Boss (1999). But for some people who live with the disorders of downward progression, communicating simply becomes too difficult, or consumes too much energy, or the person might reach a tipping point at which communicative attempts come to represent a loss of dignity and choice. When this occurs, then the matter is truly out of the clinician's hands. Strand (2003) describes this as an issue that places our beneficence—doing good for the patient—in conflict with his or her autonomy. The gifted clinician must seek a balance here, by asking and clarifying, and then backing off from encounters when the affected person chooses not to communicate.

As noted earlier, Boss's (1999) major concern is for families who witness and endure their loved ones who say goodbye without leaving. She provides many helpful suggestions for families with the uncertainties inherent in dealing with psychological absence in the face of physical presence and recently wrote a book specifically directed to helping families as they cope with dementia (Boss, 2011). The following is a list of suggestions, adapted from her work, for communication counselors working with disorders of downward progression:

- Recognize that there is no "right way" to cope with uncertainty.
- Reinforce behaviors that encourage physical activity and interaction with others.
- Encourage respite as necessary for tolerating ambiguous loss.
- Use humor as a coping mechanism.
- Guide families to harmonize with nature instead of attempting to master it.
(Boss, 1999, pp. 114–116)

The following account of the course of ALS as experienced by a client of mine serves to provide affirmation that, despite the disease, life can be lived to the end with purpose and dignity:

Mr. Luther had bulbar ALS. Soon after he was diagnosed, his wife of 50 years died suddenly of heart disease. The Luthers were childless, so Mr. Luther found himself almost alone in the world except for a sister who visited monthly and a small circle of friends. Mr. Luther, the president of a small technology company and an engineer by training, took his adversities in stride. He was a resilient person, with a passion for problem solving. Concerning his dysarthria, for example, he worked hard on developing marble-sized one-way valves to insert into his nares in hopes of reducing his increasing nasality. He could not use a standard palatal lift, so he invented one of his own, shaped like McDonald's "golden arches" and held in place by string and a button that stuck out of the corner of his mouth. Neither device worked, but he took great pleasure in creating them. (He also carried a plastic spray bottle, filled with his favorite wine, which he used liberally as his stated "best relief" both for moistening his dry mouth and for decreasing saliva.)

Frugal to a fault, as Mr. Luther's ALS worsened, he chose Magic Slates over other, more sophisticated communication devices, cutting the slates in quarters not only so they would fit comfortably in his shirt pocket but also because it saved money. He took great pains to have his affairs and his advance directives in place, making it clear to his neurologist that when he could no longer swallow, he wanted only palliative care. He also made it clear that he wanted only his sister to be with him at the end. Mr. Luther kept his autonomy until the end and accepted his impending death with grace and temperance. He said goodbye, and then made sure to leave soon thereafter.

## Positive Psychology and Disorders of Downward Progression

Does positive psychology have anything to offer? The answer is an unequivocal yes. The diagnosis of an inevitably fatal disease should not be translated immediately into "Abandon hope, all ye who enter here." Rather, it makes sense to help people with incurable diseases and their families to consider ways to live their remaining lives as fully as possible, and to help them and their families to proceed along the road of their ambiguous losses with grace and equanimity.

Joanne Koenig Coste (2003) has written a remarkably rich sourcebook for families and individuals involved in dealing with AD. Her book, *Learning to Speak Alzheimer's*, has many implications not only for the other dementias but also for most of the ambiguous losses discussed thus far. Koenig Coste names five basic tenets of habilitation, optimally applied all together in specific situations, summarized as follows:

- *Make the physical environment work.* Alter the environment in ways that help make the person feel safe, successful, comfortable, and free of distress.
- *Know that communication remains possible.* The emotions are more important than the word, and it is the emotions that need to be validated. When it's no longer possible to listen to the mouth, "listen" to the eyes.
- *Focus only on remaining skills.* Value the abilities that remain. Help the affected person to compensate without calling attention to it.
- *Live in the person's world.* Join the person in his or her current "place" or time, no matter when or where that may be, and find joy with the person there.
- *Enrich the person's life.* Create moments for success, eliminate potential moments of failure, and praise frequently and with sincerity. Attempt to find joy wherever possible.[5] (Condensed and adapted from Koenig Coste, 2003, Chapters 6–10)

Koenig Coste never uses the words "positive psychology" or "flourishing" in her book, yet she has written an affirming and fulfilling book, jammed with good ideas and suggestions for living positively with AD. Most ideas and suggestions expand on the tenets listed here. They come from her own experience in living with the disorder. Communication counselors should encourage families and individuals with dementia to read such works, preferably as early as possible in the course of the disease, so that they can apply the ideas effectively. Most of the ideas, however, have significant implications for living in institutionalized settings as well.[6]

---

[5]Dementia, particularly as it worsens, is likely to shrink the "pleasurable life" to the present, with perhaps only snatches of early past remaining and the future no longer contemplated; thus, the affected person should be helped to make the most of it—to live his or her remaining life "in the moment."

[6]The transcript of a very informative interview of Koenig Coste by the *New York Times* in 2004 is available on the Internet.

We know of Mark Reiman and his contribution to the ALS literature only because Audrey encountered his ideas on the ALS Association website (http://www.alsa.org). A treasured resource is an interview he gave 8 years after his ALS diagnosis, and 4 years before his death. Very little additional information about him is available, but his words indicate that he was a caring, measured, and brave person. The following is a list of his principles, in greatly condensed form. In essence, they constitute the framework of the counseling approach presented in this chapter.

- Seek support.
- Hold fast to hope.
- Be active in your own health.
- Realize that your life may have changed but that it's far from over.

(Adapted from Interview with Mark Reiman, 1999)

## Listening to Mark Reiman: A Positive Communication Counseling Perspective

Reiman's (Interview, 1999) principles seem comprehensive enough to serve as the springboard for elaborating on some issues in counseling persons and families experiencing disorders of downward progression. In this section, each of his points is expanded upon from the perspective of communication counseling.

### Seek Support

Early in the course of the disease, persons with disorders of downward progression can benefit from participation in groups in much the same ways as do persons with poststroke aphasia. The approach to group counseling outlined in Chapter 6 is readily applicable here.

Particularly for persons with dementia, however, group leaders will find that increased structure usually is necessary. In fact, for both group and one-on-one encounters, persons with dementia benefit from structure, limited choices, and repetition. This is in contrast to aphasic persons, who appear to flourish with freedom from them. The primary goals for such groups should be psychosocially oriented, providing opportunities to engage as fully in life as possible under changing circumstances. To capitalize on strengths, it is important to consider that early memories probably are more intact than recent ones. This includes lifelong patterns, which remain familiar as well, not only motor behaviors such as walking, or using one's native language, and the lifelong habits of doing daily chores, going to work, and being responsible.

These realities can be the basis for highly rewarding group activities. In her important resource book, *Care That Works* (1999), Zgola describes the Tea Group, a program for "difficult" [sic] residents of a long-term care (LTC) center in Ottawa, Canada, that has been in operation, despite different facilitators and members, for many years. Perhaps the goal of preparing and drinking tea is more appropriate to a committed tea-drinking country such as Canada; some adaptation may be in order for residents of the United States, where Starbucks rules. In any case, the Tea Group provides a constrained common ground, rich in habits and rituals of a lifetime, and is conducted in a safe, supportive, respectful environment that exemplifies an effective model for groups whose members have dementia.

By contrast, groups for persons with ALS or other progressive motor disorders can further the agendas of keeping as healthy as possible and preparing for change, as well as providing psychosocial support and the sharing of strengths. Many of the positive psychology interventions spread throughout this book are appropriate. Particularly for such groups, it is important to remember that for many participants, offering help as well as receiving it, is a benefit.

At least as important are partner, spouse, and family groups. The tremendous burden faced by significant others in living with and managing their partners' disorders of downward progression can be substantially influenced and lessened through group interactions. The "36-hour day" described by caregivers (Mace & Rabens, 2001) feels all too real. Caregivers need help to solve some of the problems they encounter in those long hours, as well as camaraderie and assurance that they do not bear their burdens alone.

Families of persons who have incurred strokes have similar problems, and approaches to their group counseling are similar. Using the questions in Boxes 6–4, 6–6, and 6–9, substitute the term "dementia" or "ALS" (or any of the progressive disorders) to appreciate their goodness of fit across the spectrum of these disorders.

It often is awkward and indeed disheartening for spouses of persons with PPA or the other disorders discussed here to attend groups with those whose partners have had strokes, because the courses of the disorders are fundamentally different. This is in marked contrast with the parent support groups discussed earlier, in which parents often can profit from contact with parents of children whose problems differ from those of their own children. From this perspective, it makes sense to include PPA families in dementia groups, rather than in stroke groups.

It is also possible for persons to seek and receive support without joining a formal group. The Internet, once again, can be useful, and social institutions, such as churches, can be particularly helpful.[7] Communication counselors need to familiarize themselves with programs available in their communities. For example, in Tucson, several churches provide support and respite for families with dementia, and some neighborhoods have model programs for assisting elderly and infirm persons to remain in their own homes for as long as possible.

## Hold Fast to Hope

Reiman's statement of hope (1999) is well nuanced and balanced by the acknowledgment implicit in his other principles. This is not the "cockeyed optimism" that was cautioned against earlier; rather, holding fast to hope is simply recognizing the importance of maintaining a positive attitude, even in the face of great odds. It fits well with two of Boss's tenets for managing ambiguous loss, particularly her comment that there is no right way to cope with uncertainty, and with her goal of guiding families to harmonize with nature (and its course), rather than trying to master it (Boss, 1999). Counselors who work with disorders of downward progression must be

---

[7]Recently, National Public Radio featured an interview with the Christian pop singer, Amy Grant. She spoke of the tremendous weight she felt when both of her parents, still at home, were beginning to experience dementia. She noted that she was lamenting her problems with a close friend who said, "Amy, this is the last lesson your parents are teaching you." There was a meaningful message for her in there, and for many others (including us), as well.

particularly careful not to dash the hope and optimism of clients, who may need to see things differently from their clinicians. We not only have no answers to give to them but in fact do not know how we ourselves may react in similar situations.

## Be Proactive in Health Care

Reiman reminds us that wellness is not only for the well, it can also be an attitude and a stance for the chronically, even desperately, ill. This is not a contradiction, but an affirmation about flourishing for as long as possible. Holman and Lorig (2004) and Lorig and colleagues (Lorig & Holman, 2003; Lorig, Hurwicz, Sobel, Hobbs, & Rittler, 2003) have spearheaded a self-management approach to chronic diseases such as arthritis and diabetes that has permitted affected persons to be proactive and committed to seeking wellness in the midst of their disabling conditions. John Argue (2000), an expert in movement and voice who has Parkinson disease, created a comprehensive positive exercise plan for other affected persons. The spirit of the Lee Silverman Voice Therapy approaches (LSVT Loud for SLP-As and SLVT Big for physical and occupation therapists) and their regimens lie in their allegiance to energizing and wellness (Fox, Morrison, Ramig, & Sapir, 2002). The National Center on Physical Activity and Disability (NCPAD) is committed to appropriate exercise programs for persons with deteriorating as well as stable disabling conditions and features on its website well-designed and tested programs for ALS and other degenerative motor disorders (http://www.ncpad.org). NCPAD also supports Arkin's ElderRehab program (Arkin, 1999). This program uses volunteers as aides in an effective physical exercise-language enrichment program for persons with dementia. The specifics of this program are available in a detailed resource manual (Arkin, 2005). Communication counselors need to be aware of such programs and encourage their use.

Throughout this chapter, it has been difficult to avoid use of the term "patient" to refer to these irreversibly impaired ill clients. To support a philosophy of wellness, this term is also best avoided in clinical practice. It is important for communication counselors to embrace the notion of wellness for their clients despite disability, and to encourage wellness not only for disabled adults but also for affected children and their families as well.

## Life May Be Changed, But It Is Not Over

The concept of living each day to its fullest has been emphasized throughout this book, and now it takes us back to the philosophy of Zorba the Greek, described in Chapter 1. "Full catastrophe living" most likely eludes people who are well into middle or late stages of their disorder, but it should not elude their partners and families. In this culture at least, wives are not expected to emulate their spouses' deterioration. Suttee, the practice of widows throwing themselves on their husbands' funeral pyres, is banned in India, where it once was common. It certainly should not be practiced even metaphorically in the presence of chronic illness. A particularly important point in this context is that respite from responsibility as well as maintaining humor are strong antidotes to the burdens of giving care. Not only do caregivers benefit; so do the persons for whom they are caring. Here is a pertinent story:

> When finally convinced by her clinician and her children to take a weekend trip to San Francisco with a friend, and to leave the caregiving for Mr. Y, who had moderate dementia, in the hands of her very capable daughter, Mrs. Y went reluctantly. She returned three days later, refreshed from three nights with eight hours of uninterrupted sleep, renewed by finally seeing the renovated Ferry Building about which she had heard so much, and by the gourmet meals she ate as she revisited her favorite restaurants. But there were other benefits as well. Mrs. Y learned that her daughter was a fine surrogate caregiver for short trips, that traveling with a friend produced worthy companionship and certainly more enjoyable shopping than she had ever experienced with Mr. Y, and finally, that he barely noticed her absence, and thrived on his daughter's doting. Mrs. Y began making plans for another trip three months hence.

This story was told in an AD partner group. The group had heard Mrs. Y's previous agonizing about every aspect of this trip and in fact had played a role in convincing her to go. The group members magnanimously refrained from a chorus of "We told you so," possibly because she was testing the waters for most of them as well. They could now begin the process of making plans of their own, perhaps. This is the power of support groups, which are particularly helpful in promoting the concepts of living each day as fully as possible, rather than concentrating on dying.

## Practice Your Greatest Freedom

This section begins with Mark Reiman's (Interview, 1999) exhortation to "practice your greatest freedom." He went on to offer the following advice: "Choose to make this defining moment an opportunity for your greatest love, your greatest vision, courage, determination, and compassion. Surround yourself with positive people." There is perhaps no stronger, more positive message for persons with disorders of downward progression and their families.

In Chapter 3 we pointed out that Victor Frankl believed that "choosing one's way" is the greatest freedom afforded to human beings (Frankl, 1989). Reiman explicitly acknowledges its importance in relationship to his own terminal illness. How can communication counselors help their clients to hear such a message, understand it, and apply it to their lives?

This message is not for the faint of heart, nor is it a message that can be promoted as a viable possibility to persons who do not understand it, or who do not think they can adopt it. Nonetheless, it can be shared and discussed, preferably in groups, where opinions may differ and alternatives may be explored. As an exercise, read Reiman's or Frankl's statements aloud; then check on who in the group believes this message, why it makes a difference to them, and with what beliefs it is in conflict (such as feeling victimized by one's disorder, or helpless in its presence). This message is one of life's most affirming ones, and even though not everyone can embrace it, everyone deserves a chance to consider it. Communication counselors can help make that happen.

## Counseling in Long-Term Care Settings

Thus far in this chapter, settings for intervention for the disorders of downward progression have been home based, that is, most of the clients and families who have the disorders were presumed to be living at home; however, many persons who can be managed at home only with great difficulty live in residential settings. SLPs are becoming increasingly visible in long-term care (LTC) settings.[8] By extrapolating from ASHA demographic data, it appears that roughly one quarter of all SLPs who work with adults are employed in LTCs. Audiologists are also beginning to be seen there, where they have an important part to play in enhancing the quality of life for elders who can profit from amplification. As has been true of all of the settings discussed in this book, LTC settings also offer unique opportunities and challenges.

One major counseling issue may be that of helping families reach their personally most comfortable decisions concerning placement in an LTC setting. Clearly, communication counselors seldom are the sole sources for dealing with issues such as this, but they often have an important role to play, particularly if they have been involved with management of the dementing person when he or she was still at home. The counseling skills do not change, but the focus is on helping the family and, whenever possible, the person with the disorder, to make a decision that is right for them. Koenig Coste makes a critical comment: " . . . all families will do far better when the considerations of lifespan care are dealt with on the basis of realistic assessments, rather than on guilt" (Koenig Coste, 2003, p. 192). Finally, three principles already referred to in this book should remain foremost in counseling regarding long-term placement:

1. The counselor's job is to provide options and encourage exploration of them.
2. There are neither right nor wrong decisions. There are only decisions with which one can live.
3. Decisions should reflect the values of the affected person(s), not those of the counselor.

As in rehabilitation centers, LTC administrators are increasingly encouraging staff members to work as members of interdisciplinary teams, rather than to remain isolated in the traditional

---

[8]LTC settings also may include group homes, assisted-living centers, skilled nursing facilities, nursing homes, and special care units set up in nursing homes or in assisted-living centers primarily for persons experiencing worsening dementia.

fiefdoms of nursing, occupational and physical therapy, social work, and speech-language pathology and audiology. As a result, SLP-A counseling functions are likely to be modified as well. One important new role may be as a consultant to other staff members concerning disturbed communication and nutrition, and what can be done about them. Typical in-service training sessions probably should center less on language in dementia and more on how to improve communication on site, through techniques that are taught to the staff in general, both for their own interactions with residents and to help reduce communication frustration for visitors, and on ways to promote nutrition. Some examples of LTC-centered activities developed by SLPs or occupational therapists that address each of those issues are presented next. Many more are available; all involve counseling skills to promote the most effective implementation in often fairly inflexible settings.

The Pioneer Network, in conjunction with the Centers for Medicare/Medicaid Services (CMS) is making strides in "creating home in the nursing home." One of the Network's basic concerns is to ensure that residents be allowed to make choices about "daily schedule (including when to get up, go to bed, eat, and bathe) visitation issues, homelike environment, food procurement, and so forth. All of these initiatives point directly to the counseling concerns of this book. It is important for communication counselors to be aware of these initiatives, since they all involve communication/counseling issues.

### Improving Visitor Interactions with Residents

A comprehensive booklet (Brush, 2002) is available to guide visitors in ways to improve their interactions with residents of LTCs. It is a good example of the extensive training materials available to improve daily life in LTCs. The material in this particular booklet does not need to be presented one on one; it easily stands alone. Counseling skills are involved in convincing senior staff of the value of such materials for families and indeed for anyone who interacts with residents. It offers a way to improve visits, by providing a common language and a consistent opportunity for enriching contacts for everyone. Making this happen is more likely if the SLP-A practices good counseling skills.

Finally, just as supported communication principles make sense for use with aphasia, they also are applicable with dementia. There is some overlap, to be sure, but some divergences as well. Small and colleagues' work in this area (Small, Gutman, Makela, & Hillhouse, 2003; Small & Perry, 2005) is especially instructive and applicable to both families and caregivers.

### Manipulating the Environment to Influence Nutrition and Communication in Positive Ways

A staff attuned to interdisciplinary collaborations can implement literally hundreds of environmental manipulations. The instigator may well be a communications expert, of course. Only one example is featured here, partly because it emphasizes the role of SLPs in managing nutritional issues and partly because, once again, counseling skills are not always directed at issues with residents or care providers. Here, they are employed in influencing administrative decisions. "Counseling" is not what the communication counselor does with administrators. Nevertheless, approaching such issues with counseling skills is highly recommended if changes are to be implemented.

Brush, Meehan, and Calkins (2002) described an approach to management of insufficient nutrition for residents of an LTC facility. These investigators chose a few residents who were not getting adequate nourishment and were candidates for mechanical feeding support (e.g., placement of feeding tubes). Before the experiment began, they measured participants' weight and their caloric intake, and observed their eating habits and behaviors. Two environmental manipulations followed. The first adjustment was to increase the color contrast between the table setting and the plate (both were neutral, perhaps making it difficult for residents to discern their plates and their food). The second adjustment was to increase the illumination available in the dining room setting, to increase visibility overall. During the intervention, Brush and colleagues measured caloric intake, and at its end, they weighed the participants again. Once the intervention was in place, food intake was increased; as a result, participants gained weight. Recently, building on activities such as these, this group has developed the Environmental and Communicative Protocol (ECAT, Brush, Calkins, Bruce, & Sanford,

2012).[9] Based on systematic observations, such as those described above, the ECAT is meant to identify environmental barriers to successful communication and provide ways to lessen them in long-term nursing facilities

What does all this have to do with counseling? First, to obtain permission to conduct such experimental interventions, the Brush team needed to convince the relevant administrations of the LTCs of the value of such work. Then it was necessary to ensure that the changes were carried out and to show staff the value of learning and implementing such approaches, primarily by leading them to recognize the better use of their own time. These types of messages resonate with staff and administration alike.

## Improving Staff Communication with Residents

Self-cueing and the use of cue cards in improving communication in LTC settings has been well documented (Bourgeois, Dijkstra, Burgio, & Allen-Burge, 2001; Bourgeois & Hickey, 2007). Essentially, cueing and self-cueing require SLPs to assist and teach the relevant staff to develop appropriate, situation-specific index cards that residents then can be taught to read aloud and use to cue their behaviors. For example, a certified nursing assistant (CNA) may be taught to help Mrs. T modify her repetitive questioning through the use of handwritten index cards:

> Preteaching scenario:
>
> Mrs. T: Where are my dentures?
>
> CNA: I just told you 5 minutes ago that they are being fixed and will be back next Tuesday.
>
> (This interaction may occur countless times daily.)
>
> Postteaching scenario:
>
> Mrs. T: Where are my dentures?
>
> CNA: The answer is on your card, Mrs. T. Read your card aloud.

---

[9]See Bruce, Brush, Sanford, and Calkins (2013) for data supporting ECAT's utility.

Mrs. T: [*Reads*] "My dentures are being fixed. Back on Tuesday."

CNA: Great, Mrs. T. Your dentures will be good as new next Tuesday. Next time you need to know, look at your cards.

(This interaction may occur three or four times, but practice ultimately lessens the repetitive questioning.)

The use of cue cards is a straightforward technique, as well as a simple one to teach staff. So where is the counseling involved? Communicating the method's value to the staff and demonstrating its effectiveness both require counseling skills. One facet is explicitly acknowledging the CNA's expertise. He or she probably has more knowledge of most of the residents than does the clinician-counselor. A recommended approach is to consult the CNA often, seeking partnership and demonstrating, rather than announcing, the counselor's own skills. In addition, it is wise to point out to CNAs how they may benefit from learning the approach, because it can make their jobs easier and more pleasant. Many more examples are provided in the works of Bourgeois and colleagues (2001, 2007), Koenig Coste (2003), and Zgola (1999), as well as by other writers of sourcebooks for working with dementia, such as Nissenboim and Vroman (2003). Although this book is not about management of dementia, in LTC settings the counseling roles of SLP-As often extend beyond family to other staff and support personnel.

## The Problem of Dysphagia

Dysphagia often occurs with disorders of downward progression, as well as disorders covered in Chapter 6. For many persons with swallowing disorders, substantial psychosocial issues, such as fear of choking, embarrassment over difficulty in eating unusually textured foods, and prolonged length of time required for eating, are increasingly recognized. Such issues may predispose dysphagic persons perhaps to eat alone, rather than engaging in the social interactions that accompany mealtimes. (For a cogent overview, see Martino, 2005.) These problems pull dysphagia into mainstream communications counseling and do not necessarily require specialized counseling expertise. Nevertheless, such concerns truly demand our attention. An exciting development concerning the question of LTC food management has recently been described by Bowman (2013). She discusses new dining practice guidelines developed by the previously mentioned Pioneer Network/CMS alliance and approved by a large number of relevant professional organizations, including ASHA. These new guidelines should overcome many of the barriers that negatively affect our ability to advocate for, and to effectively address, the aforementioned issues in food management for LTC residents.

When dysphagia is life threatening to the person whose disorder is worsening, such as in ALS, or when the affected person may not understand all the issues, as in dementia, the placement of feeding tubes becomes both a compelling issue for families and a great challenge for communication counselors. Irwin (2006) noted that SLPs often play an important role not only in counseling but also in advising others who may be providing counseling about the placement of feeding tubes. Irwin was specifically discussing dementing persons whose conditions had deteriorated to dependence on feeding tubes for maintenance of life, but many of his points are also relevant to persons with advanced ALS. In light of limited data on the effectiveness of feeding tubes for preventing aspiration (Chouinard, Lavigne, & Villeneuve, 1998; Dharmarajan & Unnikrishnan, 2004; Finucane, Christmas, & Travis, 1999), SLPs face dilemmas about how to advise family members, even when advance directives are already in place. (Irwin notes a startling finding by Shega, Hougham, Stocking, Cox-Hayley, and Sachs, 2003, indicating that 36% of physicians would place a feeding tube at a family's request, despite advance directives to the contrary.) Other studies indicate that both SLPs and physicians often have incomplete information about the limited effectiveness of feeding tubes (Carey, 2005; Conti, 2003).

Listening to families and helping them to clarify such issues, providing them with significant and valid information to aid them in making decisions regarding feeding tubes, and the like, are counseling functions. As Irwin (2006) suggests, however, that appropriate counseling requires professionals who have a predominantly rehabilitative outlook to shift their outlook to a palliative one. This means essentially shifting attention toward an attitude of "active total care of patients whose condition is not responsive to curative treatment," as defined in 1990 by the World Health Organization (WHO). Box 7–2 provides the WHO's complete definition of palliative care.

---

**Box 7–2. Dimensions of Palliative Care**

- Affirms life and regards dying as a normal process
- Neither hastens nor postpones death
- Provides relief from pain and other distressing symptoms
- Offers a support system to help patients live as actively as possible until death
- Offers a support system to help the family cope during the patient's illness and in their own bereavement

(From World Health Organization, 2001.)

---

## Are All LTC Facilities Created Equal?

Both good LTC facilities and barely passable ones (at least from the above perspective) can be certified despite their differences in philosophy, quality and range of services, and outlook. Communication counselors may well find themselves in the role of giving information to families about the quality of the institutions they are considering, listening to their concerns, and guiding them in their choices. Koenig Coste (2003) provides sensible guidelines for families to follow. The list of guidelines gets longer as the need for services increases from assisted living to special dementia units. Koenig Coste stresses that few LTC facilities, even at the assisted-living level, meet all expectations, but it is nonetheless worthwhile to consider these guidelines from a personal standpoint, looking for the facility that comes closest to the family's ideal. Her basic guidelines for assisted living appear in condensed form in Box 7–3.

One recognized approach to LTC has been developed by The Eden Alternative, a community-based model that focuses on maximizing quality of life for both residents and workers in LTC facilities.

According to the Eden Alternative website, this model is dedicated to creating "coalitions of people and organizations that are committed to creating better social and physical environments for people." From the perspective of positive psychology, it is difficult

> ### Box 7–3. Things to Look for
> ### When Selecting a Long-Term Care Facility
>
> - Is the location convenient for regular visits?
> - Can you drop in for a tour any time or does the management insist on guiding it?
> - Will the resident be safe from the dangers of wandering?
> - Is the staff specifically trained for interactions with persons who have dementia?
> - Does the staff appear to enjoy interacting with residents?
> - Is the pervasive odor a good one?
> - Are common areas well designed and inviting?
> - Are residents encouraged to personalize their rooms?
> - Are the activity programs of interest to the residents?
> - Are there opportunities and areas for outdoor activities?
> - Does the center involve families in formulating its plan of care?
> - Is the food appetizing, nutritious, and suitable for the declining skills of the residents?
> - Will the faculty provide names and contact information for references from other families?
> - If dementing residents intermingle with other residents, are they treated with friendliness and support?
>
> ---
>
> (Adapted from Koenig Coste, 2003.)

to imagine a more appropriate LTC facility than one grounded in Eden Alternative principles, presented in Box 7–4. Such LTC facilities are flourishing across the United States. SLP-As who are considering working in extended care settings may find these principles useful as a gauge against which to judge an environment in which they wish to work.[10]

---

[10]A recent article by Rebecca Mead (2013, May 20) in *The New Yorker* describes another example of person-centered dementia care, the Beatitudes Campus Retirement Community in Phoenix, Arizona. The article provides a good introduction to this growing trend that also includes the previously mentioned Pioneer Network.

## Box 7–4. Eden Alternative Principles

1. The three plagues of loneliness, helplessness, and boredom account for the bulk of suffering among our Elders.

2. An Elder-centered community commits to creating a Human Habitat where life revolves around close and continuing contact with plants, animals and children. It is these relationships that provide the young and old alike with a pathway to a life worth living.

3. Loving companionship is the antidote to loneliness. Elders deserve easy access to human and animal companionship.

4. An Elder-centered community creates opportunity to give as well as receive care. This is the antidote to helplessness.

5. An Elder-centered community imbues daily life with variety and spontaneity by creating an environment in which unexpected and unpredictable interactions and happenings can take place. This is the antidote to boredom.

6. Meaningless activity corrodes the human spirit. The opportunity to do things that we find meaningful is essential to human health.

7. Medical treatment should be the servant of genuine human caring, never its master.

8. An Elder-centered community honors its Elders by de-emphasizing top-down bureaucratic authority, seeking instead to place the maximum possible decision-making authority into the hands of the Elders or into the hands of those closest to them.

9. Creating an Elder-centered community is a never-ending process. Human growth must never be separated from human life.

10. Wise leadership is the lifeblood of any struggle against the three plagues. For it, there can be no substitute.

_____

(From The Eden Alternative, 2002.)

## Conclusion

As supported by this chapter, counseling and coaching are at least as much an attitude and a state of mind as they are a set of skills brought to bear on a problem of interest. In Chapter 3 we discussed the importance of identifying detrimental personal attitudes and maintaining respect for those whom we counsel. Attitude seems pervasive in relation to the disorders focused on here. Perhaps this is because our roles with these disorders are less clear and, particularly with dementia, have only recently been recognized as important.

Irwin (2006) was astute in describing our optimal role with dysphagia in late-stage dementia, or with ventilator placement in late-stage ALS, as palliative, rather than rehabilitative. His observation should be extended, however, to include *all* disorders of downward progression: Palliation is the indicated approach in each of these disorders. Accordingly, communication counseling is central to all of our interactions and engagements with affected persons, their families, and staff members of the facilities where they may ultimately reside.

Koenig Coste has had infinitely more direct experience with disorders of downward progression, or at least in dementia, than most people. Her earliest encounter with AD occurred well over 30 years ago when her husband (somewhat older than she) was first suspected of having it, while she was pregnant with their fourth child. From her story, it appears that she embraced the disorder, accepting its challenges and its inevitable changes, and, upon the death of her husband, moved toward it. Instead of closing the door on that chapter of her life, she found her life's work in learning more about AD, as well as in sharing her personal experiences with others who find themselves in the same boat. Even today, her attitudes and her creativity remain intact, and she has not suffered the burnout reported by many people who work with these disorders. Whatever Koenig Coste's particular character strengths may be, certainly bravery and vitality must be high on the list.

Koenig Coste may well be the Johnny Appleseed of AD, sharing her compassion, ideas, and knowledge with those who need it most, and carrying forward the wisdom she also has gained from others. It seems appropriate to end this chapter with her observations on how persons with dementia can best be supported to live well:

- Reminding and scolding me does not make me better, only sadder. When someone asks me questions about where I've been and who I've seen and what I did, and I can't retrieve that information, I feel stupid and unworthy.
- Trying to fill my brain with new ideas and new equipment and new data will not work. My brain is full. Not one speck of space is left for new information to find a seat. If the information can't go in, it can never come out again.
- Don't wish me out of reverie or worry about my silent times. I still have imaginative explorations to make, and dreams to dream. I have kisses to relive. I have a garden of memories before me, and everything is blooming simultaneously. Don't assume I am sad when I sit alone; most of the time it is the sadness on your face that brings sorrow to my heart.
- You can make me a part of this world only if you actively involve me, if your connection with me remains until the end. You must constantly reach out and touch me—physically, spiritually, emotionally.
- You are the conduit to my failing world, a world that has so many possibilities to be filled with laughter, a few shared tears, and memories.
(From Koenig Coste, 2003, pp. 198–199)

These words apply to persons with all varieties of dementias and, perhaps with the exception of the second point, to all of the others whose disorders involve saying goodbye without leaving, as well.

## References

Argue, J. (2000). *Parkinson's disease and the art of moving*. Oakland, CA: New Harbinger.

Arkin, S. (1999). ElderRehab: A student-supervised exercise program for Alzheimer's patients. *Gerontologist, 39,* 729–735.

Arkin, S. (2005). *Language enriched exercise for clients with Alzheimer's disease.* Tucson, AZ: Desert Fitness.

Bayles, K., & Tomoeda, C. (2007). *Cognitive-communication disorders of dementia: Definition, diagnosis, and treatment.* San Diego, CA: Plural.

Beauby, J.-C. (1998). *The diving bell and the butterfly.* New York, NY: Vintage Press.

Boss, P. (1999). *Ambiguous loss: Learning to live with unresolved grief.* Cambridge, MA: Harvard University Press.

Boss, P. (2011). *Loving someone who has dementia hope when caring: How to find hope while coping with stress and grief.* San Francisco, CA: Jossey-Bass.

Bourgeois, M., Dijkstra, K., Burgio, L., & Allen-Burge, R. (2001). Memory aids as an AAC strategy for nursing home residents with dementia. *Augmentative and Alternative Communication, 17,* 196–210.

Bourgeois, M., & Hickey, E. (2007). Dementia. In D. Beukelman, K. Garrett, & K. Yorkston (Eds.), *Communication strategies for adults with acute or chronic medical conditions.* Baltimore, MD: Paul H. Brookes.

Bourgeois, M., & Hickey, E. (2009). *Dementia: From diagnosis to management. A functional approach.* New York, NY: Taylor & Francis.

Bowman, C. (2013). Ten new dining practice standards: Speech-language pathologists guide to their implementation. *Seminars in Speech and Language, 34*(1), 37–41.

Bruce, C., Brush, J., Sanford, J., & Calkins, M. (2013). Development and evaluation of the Environment and Communication Toolkit (ECAT) with speech-language pathologists. *Seminars in Speech and Language, 34*(1), 42–51.

Brush, J. (Ed.). (2002). *Ideas for a better visit.* Kirtland, OH: Ideas Institute.

Brush, J., Calkins, M., Bruce, C., & Sanford, J. (2012). *Environment and communication assessment toolkit for dementia care.* Baltimore, MD: Health Professions Press.

Brush, J. A., Meehan, R. A., & Calkins, M. P. (2002). Using the environment to improve intake in people with dementia. *Alzheimer's Care Quarterly, 3*(4), 330–338.

Carey, T. S. (2005). Use of feeding tubes in the care of long-term residents. *North Carolina Medical Journal, 66,* 313–315.

Chouinard, J., Lavigne, E., & Villeneuve, C. (1998). Weight loss, dysphagia, and outcome in advanced dementia. *Dysphagia, 13,* 151–155.

Conti, G. (2003). Speech-language pathologists' role and knowledge levels related to non-oral feeding. *Journal of Medical Speech-Language Pathology, 11,* 15–31.

Dharmarajan, T., & Unnikrishnan, D. (2004). Tube feeding in the elderly: The technique, complications and outcome. *Postgraduate Medicine, 115,* 51–54, 58–61.

Finucane, T., Christmas, C., & Travis, K. (1999). Tube feeding in patients with advanced dementia: A review of the evidence. *Journal of the American Medical Association, 282,* 1365–1370.

Fox, C., Morrison, C., Ramig, L., & Sapir, S. (2002). Current perspectives on the Lee Silverman Voice Treatment (LSVT®). *American Journal of Speech Language Pathology, 11,* 111–123.

Frankl, V. (1989). *Man's search for meaning.* New York, NY: Washington Square Press.

Irwin, W. (2006). Feeding patients with advanced dementia: The role of the speech-language pathologist in making end-of-life decisions. *Journal of Medical Speech-Language Pathology, 14,* xi–xiii.

Holman, A., & Lorig, K. (2004). Patient self-management: A key to effectiveness and efficiency in care of chronic disease. *Public Health Reports, 119,* 239–243.

Koenig Coste, J. (2003). *Learning to speak Alzheimer's: A groundbreaking approach for everyone dealing with the disease.* Boston, MA: Houghton Mifflin.

Lorig, K., & Holman, H. (2003). Self-management education: History, definition outcomes and mechanisms. *Annals of Behavioral Medicine, 26,* 1–7.

Lorig, K., Hurwicz, M., Sobel, D., Hobbs, M., & Rittler, P. (2003). A national dissemination of an evidence based self-management program: A process evaluation study. *Patient Education and Counseling, 1,* 69–79.

Mace, N. L., & Rabens, P. V. (2001). *The 36-hour day: A family guide to caring for persons with Alzheimer disease, related dementing illnesses, and memory loss in later life.* Baltimore, MD: Johns Hopkins University Press.

Martino, R. (2005). Food for thought: Does what the patient thinks really matter? *Perspectives on Swallowing and Swallowing Disorders (Dysphagia). Division 13 Newsletter of the American Speech-Language-Hearing Association, 14*(4), 24–26.

Mead, R. (2013, May 20). The sense of an ending. *The New Yorker.*

Nissenboim, S., & Vroman, C. (2003). *The positive interactions program of activities for people with Alzheimer's disease.* Baltimore, MD: Health Professions Press.

Rippon, G. A., Scarmeas, N., Gordon, P. H., Murphy, P. L., Albert, S. M., Mitsumoto, H., . . . Stern, Y. (2006). An observational study of cognitive impairment in amyotrophic lateral sclerosis. *Archives of Neurology, 63,* 345–352.

Rogers, M. A., King, J., & Alarcon, N. B. (2000). Proactive management of primary progressive aphasia. In D. R. Beukelman, K. Yorkston, & J. Reichle (Eds.), *Augmentative communication for adults with neuro-*

genic and neuromuscular disabilities (pp. 305–337). Baltimore, MD: Paul H. Brookes.

Shega, J., Hougham, G. W., Stocking, C., Cox-Hayley, D., & Sachs, G. (2003). Barriers to limiting the practice of feeding tube placement in advanced dementia. *Journal of Palliative Medicine, 6,* 885–893.

Small, J., Gutman, G., Makela, S., & Hillhouse, B. (2003). Effectiveness of communication strategies used by caregivers of persons with Alzheimer's disease during activities of daily living. *Journal of Speech, Language, and Hearing Research, 46,* 353–367.

Small, J., & Perry, J. (2005). Do you remember? How caregivers question their spouses who have Alzheimer's disease and the impact on communication. *Journal of Speech, Language, and Hearing Research, 48,* 125–136.

Strand, E. (2003). Clinical and professional ethics in the management of motor speech disorders. *Seminars in Speech and Language, 24,* 301–311.

World Health Organization. (2001). Definition of palliative care. In C. F. von Gunten, F. D. Ferris, R. K. Portenoy, & M. Glajchen (Eds.), *CAPC manual* (online publication). New York, NY: Center to Advance Palliative Care. Retrieved from http://64.85.16.230/educate/content/palliative caredefinitions/WHO

Zgola, J. (1999). *Care that works.* Baltimore, MD: Johns Hopkins Press.

## Websites

National Institute of Neurological Disorders and Stroke ALS website: http://www.ninds.nih.gov; follow links to "Disorders" and then "Amyotrophic Lateral Sclerosis"

ALS Association: http://www.alsa.org

Alzheimer's Association: http://www.alz.org

Alzheimer's Foundation of America: http://www.Alzfdn.org

National Center on Physical Activity and Disability: http://www.ncpad.org

National Institutes of Health Senior Health Health Information for Older Adults: http://www.nihseniorhealth.gov

Pioneer Network: http://www.pioneer.net

Also check YouTube offerings frequently for relevant videos. Some videos that are particularly noteworthy concerning dementia are as follows:

"I remember better when I paint" French Connection Film (Hilgos Foundation)

"What's that? (English language version, Movie Teller films)

YouTube™ clips from the Alive Inside Project (Daniel Cohen, MSW)

# Chapter 8

# TEACHING RESILIENCE AND OPTIMISM TO FAMILIES AND PERSONS WITH COMMUNICATION DISORDERS: SOME WORKSHOP FORMATS

## Introduction

Scattered throughout this book are suggestions for counseling moments and exercises that foster adaptation, growth, and the development of positive attitudes concerning communication impairments and their consequences. To this point, it has been assumed that they would be applied within the traditional formats for individual and group treatments in speech-language pathology and audiology. This chapter describes an additional model: short-term workshops specifically targeting the importance of resilience, optimism, and positive attitudes for persons who have communication disorders and their families, partners, and parents, as applicable. Some activities for these proposed workshops have been discussed in previous chapters; they are revisited briefly in this new format. Other activities are presented here for the first time. Just as many of the previously described activities can fit into a short-term workshop model, the new ones can be used in more standard individual and group treatment sessions.

## Format and Background for the Workshops

The short-term workshops described here each consist of four sessions, 1.5 to 2 hours in length, spread over four consecutive weeks. This time frame works well for the busy schedules of many clients and professionals, although other formats can be used. The activities can very easily be spread over more sessions (say, six) or over longer periods (say, meetings every two weeks), or perhaps concentrated into an all-day workshop. This last format precludes the advantage that spacing provides, namely, that participants have an opportunity to try out the material, report back, and make it possible for the facilitator to debrief or help to correct, if necessary. The workshops can also be considerably expanded. The suggested activities are not cast in concrete, either. They are merely suggestions, chosen from a much wider array of potential activities, either because some have data to support their effectiveness or because in our clinical practice they have been especially useful with persons who have communication disorders.

The workshops are designed for any number of participants. Although the frameworks for, say, 10 attendees would be more personalized than they would be for larger groups, the principles do not vary. For example, if the workshop is small, then during the first session everyone probably will be able to share experiences; this will certainly not be possible with 30 or more participants.

Workshops for parents of at-risk children probably can be broad, and families can learn from others with different problems quite successfully. But there is no inherent problem in directing a workshop toward a specific disability, such as autism or Down syndrome. The suggested reading lists and websites may vary with the focus topic, but little else. Workshops for older children and adolescents who stutter or who have incurred traumatic brain injury (TBI) probably should be disorder specific, particularly if bonding and reaching out are to be emphasized. Severity of the disorder should provide guidelines as well.

Positively oriented workshops for adults and their families are different. These workshops probably should always be disorder focused. Although the workshop principles do not differ, and in many cases, the activities also are similar, mutual support and bonding are less likely to be effective if persons with aphasia and right hemisphere brain damage (RHD) or TBI, or their families, participate in the same sessions, or when persons with dementia and those with disorders such as amyotrophic lateral sclerosis (ALS) are grouped. This is largely because the challenges of these disorders differ markedly.

This chapter provides communication counselors with an alternative framework for helping their clients begin to discern the benefits to be gained by practicing some of the principles espoused in this book. It is not a blueprint for conducting such workshops; it is merely a set of workable ideas. Neither are four sessions like these likely to change the course of anyone's life.[1] Nevertheless, such workshops may constitute the first step along such a path. They can provide common ground for future counseling; they also can serve as the necessary stimulus for participants to follow through with self-directed activities such as reading and applying relevant, lay-oriented materials such as in Reivich and Shatté's book (2002), or involving themselves through the Authentic Happiness website (http://www.authentichappiness.com) or lay readings described earlier, or in taking the online courses based on the work of Reivich and Shatté. (Again, the online courses can be accessed through http://www.reflectivelearning.com.)

This chapter contains workshop outlines for parents of children with disabilities, and for families of adults who have incurred communication disorders. For the parent workshops, no particular

---

[1]In fact, it is not even particularly likely that at the end of the workshops, direct or potentially long-lasting effects will be found. In a workshop based on this model that Audrey conducted with persons with acquired immunodeficiency syndrome, supportive bonds were formed that have continued. But the real value is reflected in a comment made a year later by a member of the group, who said that the workshop had been the impetus for a year of personal exploration and change (including breaking his previously unbreakable addiction to cigarettes).

disorder has been specified, since getting together parents of children who have different disabilities can be a plus.

For the family workshop, activities are focused on families (spouses, partners, children) of disabled adults, occasionally using some specific disorder as illustrative. Some topics and exercises for parents and family differ only in their details (where the devil has been said to reside), but some are unique to each target group. Nevertheless, the basic information can be generalized to other family or disorder groups, such as Parkinson disease or Alzheimer disease (AD), as well as to parent groups aimed at specific disorders such as autism or Down syndrome.

A review of communication counselors' preparation for conducting these workshops follows. Then the parent and family workshops are presented in detail. Finally, ideas concerning how they may be modified for use with adolescent stutterers and with persons with aphasia are explored. These latter workshop variations are described only briefly, owing to the overlap with the family and parent approaches.

## Workshop Preparation for Communication Counselors

If you are still reading this book, then it is obvious that it is a recommended text. Nonetheless, other very useful readings can help you prepare for conducting workshops of this nature. Many references from other chapters constitute excellent background material, particularly Seligman's books, *Authentic Happiness* (2002) and *Flourish* (2011); Peterson's *A Primer in Positive Psychology* (2006); and Reivich and Shatté's *The Resilience Factor: Seven Essential Skills for Overcoming Life's Inevitable Obstacles* (2002). Once again, Heath and Heath's *Switch* (2010) is also excellent reading, not only for the person giving workshops of this nature, but for families as well.

Performance of at least one "dress rehearsal" of this workshop is recommended before implementation with the relevant group. A simple way to practice is with colleagues, or students, or even a group of persons with communication disorders or their families with whom you have had extensive and positive contact, and who can be counted on to provide constructive feedback. (Many of these "guinea pigs" will find the workshops interesting and useful in their own lives.)

The cardinal difference between workshops and more traditional group sessions is that workshops frequently attempt to teach new skills or to reach new understandings based on new learning. They typically incorporate information giving, in the form of informal lecturing, as well as through interaction among the group's participants. These workshops are no exceptions. Nonetheless, even though new information is emphasized, the basic commitment to shared expertise should be respected. This means that group leaders must recognize the importance of their listening role as well as their talking role. Group leaders facilitate learning along with the experience of putting the concepts and the exercises into practice. The experiences and the group's discussion of them are central. It often is worth skimping on the informal lecturing for the sake of just jumping into it.

In many cases, the exercises for the parent and family versions overlap. When they do not, both a parent and a family variant are provided. Note that all of these exercises and homework instructions are presented as simply springboards for counselors' own creative adaptations. Incidentally, the terms *counselor, facilitator, leader,* and *communication counselor* are used interchangeably in this chapter.

## Week 1

One of the workshop leader's first responsibilities is to let the participants know what they can expect to learn and experience, and what is expected of them. The purpose of this initial session is to jumpstart that process, and to get participants acquainted with one another as they begin to share solutions and strengths, and to provide support for one another.

### The First Activity: A Positive Start

An effective way to initiate these workshops is the "You at Your Best" example presented in Chapter 2. Box 8–1 contains a modification

---

**Box 8–1. Week 1: You at Your Best—Workshop Format**

*Instructions:* Think of a time in your life when you were at your very best. Then write a brief description of the event and what you did that showed you at your best. It does not have to be a long description, perhaps just some notes on it. Limit yourself to 10 minutes for the entire exercise.

Now find someone you do not know in this room. Go sit with that person, and tell each other your stories. This should take about 10 min.

---

that has been used successfully for this purpose. It serves both as an experiential introduction to positive psychology and as an excellent first step in building new relationships. During the exercise, a lot of noise and laughter can be expected. It is important to point this out when it happens, and to expand on it in the general discussion, as described later.

Following story sharing, the group leader then asks a participant whose partner told a very good story to share it with the group. Depending on the time, the leader may ask two or three people to tell their partner's stories. Some good questions for initiating the general discussion include the following: "What strengths were you using?" "How else do you use that strength?" The facilitator may wish to mention that the group will explore the subject of such strengths more deeply later.

Focusing this first discussion on the point that there is joy and laughter, however brief for most people, despite life's burdens, brings a lighter, generally positive note to the workshop experience. By contrast, imagine beginning a workshop for parents or families by asking people to share one significant problem faced by them or their child or aphasic family member—the tone would be quite different, with a much more solemn outcome. Seligman (2002) noted that our bad experiences are like Velcro in that they seem to stick to us; our positive ones slip away as if they were coated in Teflon. Putting one's best foot forward often is awkward for people because of the "Velcro effect," and is a good discussion point as well. Other discussion points may include the importance of sharing stories with others and how such sharing furnishes an interesting counterweight to the common tendency to focus on problems, rather than on successes.

## The Second Activity:  Participant Introductions

The second activity of this session is to make sure that participants begin the process of getting to know each other. Participants are each asked to say why they are here, to introduce themselves briefly, and also briefly to describe their child or the family member. Depending on group size, such disclosure can be more or less detailed. The leader's initial job is to model the introduction in his or her own identifying comments and then monitor the time, provide organizing remarks, and finally summarize shared and unique experiences, common themes, and the like.

## Introducing Positive Psychology

The introduction to positive psychology should be as brief and as informal as possible. Chapter 2 provides a good starting place. It is useful to cast the information into a form that considers the questions, "Why do some parents or families or individuals with aphasia seem to cope better than others?" or "What does it take to be resilient?" Then the facilitator can discuss the idea that the science of positive psychology examines questions like these and has begun to provide some answers. For example, the following attributes describe families or parents who do well:

- Understand the three paths to authentic happiness
- Know their strengths
- See alternatives
- Have an optimistic attitude, tempered by realism
- Know how to use, or to counteract, their explanatory styles
- Have "bounce back" and "muddle through" skills
- Know when and where to seek help.

The goal is not to explain positive psychology in any depth but simply to let parents or families know that they will be learning some skills and techniques during the course of the workshop that will be useful in launching them in an affirming direction.

## The Third Activity: Character Strengths and Virtues

The final activity of the first session is to participate in the card-shuffle version of the character strengths and virtues activity described in Chapter 6. The version presented there was for use with aphasic adults, but it is easily adaptable here for parents or families as well. Some suggestions for group discussion after completion of this activity are given in Box 8–2.

## Homework

Homework is an integral part of this workshop model. Homework helps to ensure that the ideas discussed during each session go

---

### Box 8–2. Week 1: Signature-Strengths Card Shuffle—Sample Discussion Questions

- Are your five top cards all the same color? What do you think that means?
- What do you think it might mean if they are all different colors?
- Was it easy to find cards that describe you? Did you have more than five?
- Which is the biggest of your stacks? ("Like me," "Not like me," or "?")
- From your "Like me" stack, which one describes you best? With which do you feel most comfortable?

*For parents:*

Did that strength help you since your child was born? How? Is it helping you now?

*For family members:*

Did that strength help you since your spouse's (or partner's or parent's) illness? How? Is it helping you now?

beyond the session's confines to practical application at home. Reivich points out that homework provides an opportunity to take the ideas presented in a workshop for a "test drive" so that subsequent sessions can focus on what was successful and what was not (K. Reivich, personal communication, 2006).

It is a good idea to provide small spiral notebooks to participants so that they can record their experiences in doing the assignments. An alternative is to provide formatted assignment sheets that summarize the exercises and provide space for writing a summary of the experience. Box 8–3 describes the first homework task, a set of extensions of the "You at Your Best" activity. Workshop participants are asked to try to do at least one of these assignments, or perhaps more. Please note that "your child" is purposely ambiguous. These suggestions can easily apply to any of your children, not just the one who is the focus of this workshop

The second homework assignment is to reconsider a strength that each participant has identified through the card-shuffle exercise, and to use that strength in a new way during the week before the next workshop session.[2] This exercise, described in Chapter 2 in relation to the formal VIA questionnaire, is easily adaptable here.

---

### Box 8–3. Week 1: Homework—Everybody at His or Her Best in the Everyday World

*Parent version:*

- Think of a time when you were at your very best with your child. Then write a brief description of the event and what you did that showed you at your best.
- Think of a time when your partner was at his or her very best with your child. Then write a brief description of the event and what he or she did.

---

[2]As noted earlier, Peterson (2006, pp. 159–162) presents a long list of ideas concerning how to do this.

■ Think of a time when one of your other children was at his or her very best with the child who is the focus of this workshop. Then write a brief description of the event and what he or she did.

■ Think of a time when your child was at his or her very best. Then write a brief description of the event, and what your child did.

Clearly, nobody will do all of these assignments within a week, but they are important to ponder. Try to write at least a few words for yourself (possibly to share with the group) about the first and last points. Revisit the exercise as often as possible, if only in your thoughts.

*Family version:*

■ Think of a time when you were at your very best with your family member. Then write a brief description of the event and what you did that showed you at your best.

■ Think of a time when your family member recently was at his or her very best with you. Then write a brief description of the event and what he or she did. Does it compare in any way with the person at his or her very best *before* the disabling event?

■ Think of a time when another family member was at his or her very best with the family member who is the focus of this workshop. Then write a brief description of the event and what he or she did.

Again, clearly, nobody will do all of these assignments within a week, but they are important to ponder. Try to write at least a few words for yourself (possibly to share with the group) about the first two points. Revisit the exercise whenever you need. Note that the use of "family member" is as ambiguous as the use of "the child" above.

Even when participants have not completed these assignments, most report that they have at least thought about the assignments. (This also can be a subsequent discussion focus, that is, what makes the exercises hard for some people to do?)

# Week 2

As will be the pattern for the rest of the workshop sessions, the second session starts by sharing the lessons learned and some of the experiences that occurred in carrying out the assignments. It is unreasonable to expect that all workshop participants will complete all assignments, but some will. They will have stories to tell that are informative not only to other participants who did the assignments but also to those who did not. Here is a good place to find out what may make exercises hard for some participants. It also is a good place to ask the "non-doers" (gently) if the experiences that any of the doers reported were useful to them. This is a time for story sharing, and as in the previous session, the leader's role is to monitor time, to point out themes, and so forth, and to summarize what the group members have discovered about themselves or others.

## Defining and Discussing Resilience

The second session then explores what resilience is, and why it is important to learn and practice resilience skills. This is a crucial point for parents who are raising challenging children, or for families who are living with a disabled adult. A handout for this session could be the list of characteristics of Vietnam prisoners of war who did *not* develop posttraumatic stress disorder as presented in Box 2–2. It is important to point out that becoming more resilient is possible; one's ability to bounce back, or to steer through, or simply to take life in stride is not immutable. Change and growth are possible.

There are a lot of resilience skills and strategies, as well as many ways to practice and then to incorporate them into daily life (some are listed in Chapter 2, but see Reivich and Shatté, 2002, for a fuller list). These skills are closely related. The following four skills probably are most immediately accessible to parents and families:[3]

---

[3]You may wish to choose others, but the point is to provide exercises that you believe illustrate simple resilience techniques that can be profitably applied to and by almost anyone.

- Learning the importance of taking risks
- Recognizing and regulating emotions—comprising two components: learning to identify feelings and then learning to control one's emotional responses to events and situations
- Learning to trust oneself, to count on one's strengths, and to develop a sense of mastery
- Learning the importance of reaching out to others.

Each of these skills is discussed briefly next.

## Risk Taking

For many people, simply attending a workshop amounts to taking a risk; thus, no special exercise is suggested, and in its place, the concept of taking risks and its importance in living with disabilities serves as the first discussion topic. The facilitator may begin the session by noting that the participants were not ordered to come to these sessions, nor were any promises made about the workshop's outcome—yet here they are, in what (before the last session at least) was a step, if not a full-fledged leap, into an unknown experience. Some potential questions for the discussion include the following:

- Why did you come?
- What are your expectations?
- What risks did you take just to be here?
- How does stepping off into the unknown relate to having children with disabilities? To living with adults who have them?
- Is taking risks a necessity?
- What risks have you taken? In general? In relation to your child or family member?
- What does risk taking have to do with resilience?

A discussion of questions such as these leads directly into some exercises designed to illustrate resilience and to practice some of its skills.

## Activity One: Recognizing and Regulating Emotions

The "Recognizing and Regulating Emotions" exercise is designed to help participants gain control of emotional responses in stressful personal interactions and events. Every life has stressors, but ample evidence indicates that they are disproportionate for parents and families living with disability. There are many ways to deal with stress, but common to most of them are calming techniques, ranging from taking a few deep breaths, to learning to manage breathing, to systematic progressive relaxation. These *stepping back* approaches permit the person experiencing stress to take stock of the situation and attempt to put it into perspective. This workshop provides practice for a simple and quite effective approach, similar to the pauses discussed in Chapter 3 and as important for communication counselors to learn to use before replying to clients.

Workshop participants are taught a set of specific techniques to use in handling a negative stressful event: (1) Immediately identify and name the feeling, that is, identify the initial emotional response.[4] (2) Then, before responding, take a deep breath, instruct yourself to calm down, and wait for 20 seconds. During that time, think of alternative responses—it does not matter, at this point, whether these alternative responses are positive or negative. (3) Then re-evaluate the initial reaction, and perhaps modify it before responding by word or action.

This takes practice, but fortunately all the practice does not have to be on the firing line. All of us have experienced stressful situations when we wish we had reacted differently, and one form of practice is to mentally replay some of those old instances and imagine a different response. It also can be instructive to read advice columns in the newspaper. Because the content of the letters and responses typically is emotionally charged, an interesting exercise is to register one's emotions and responses while reading the column and then compare them with the recommendations of "Dear Abby" or another columnist. Another approach is to practice with scenarios. Box 8–4 contains four examples: two for parents and two for families.

---

[4]You may wish to begin this exercise by having the group provide names for a variety of negative emotions, such as fear, anger, guilt, jealousy, or disappointment.

**Box 8–4. Week 2: Exercise for
Recognizing and Regulating Emotions**

The group leader reads a scenario and asks participants to write down their emotional responses, immediately, before thinking about it. Then the leader asks participants to think about their responses and come up with some alternatives. Each scenario is discussed in turn, with volunteers from the group contributing their suggestions. Relevant questions may include the following:

- Why is it important to recognize and control emotional responses?
- Once you have practiced it for a while, how can you pass this skill on to other members of the family (including your children)?

*Parent version:*

1. Your 9-year-old daughter was crying when she got off the school bus. She reported that three other girls from the neighborhood had teased her "all the way home" because she came from the special class. They also told her, she says, that she was "funny looking."
2. You and your wife have been researching cochlear implants for your 6-month-old son, Victor, who has a severe hearing impairment According to some of the extensive material you have read, implantation can occur as early as 12 months. You both are eager to have the surgery as soon as possible. You schedule a visit to the cochlear implant clinic in the medical center closest to your home, where Victor is evaluated. Both the pediatric otolaryngologist and the audiologist tell you that they cannot be sure at this point that Victor is a candidate, and that in any event, they will not consider implementation until he is reevaluated at age 2 years.

*Family version:*

1. Your aphasic family member's most vexing problem since his stroke is that he has not been permitted to drive again.

You are not very happy about it either, because you must now do all the driving. Your physician finally gives you permission to seek out a retraining program for handicapped drivers. You schedule an appointment with the driving training person, and when you arrive, she tells you that she does not train people with language problems because she does not believe that they can be counted on to drive safely.

2. You and your spouse have always been part of a traditional family Thanksgiving dinner that rotates from home to home in your extensive family. Your sister, who is this year's hostess, tells you that it would be "better for all" if you did not bring your wife, who has moderate AD, to this year's dinner, "because it makes everyone so sad to see her that way."

### Activity Two:  Learning to Trust Yourself

*Self-efficacy* is the fancy word for trusting yourself, knowing your strengths and how you can use them to cope with adversity and to solve problems. Few people believe they can handle every task, although most are pretty sure of their ability to come through in some. The hard ones are the tough situations, but if they look at self-mastery overall, people are likely to see their character strengths shining through. Audrey's experience furnishes an illustration:

I happen to have Angel Food Cake Self-Efficacy (AFCSE). With the level of competence I have managed to attain, I trust myself to produce a perfect cake every time (well, *most* every time!). A look back on how I achieved AFCSE showed a combination of contributing factors: (1) It took practice; (2) it happened in small steps, not all at once; and (3) it was notably enhanced by using my signature strengths—humor, curiosity, and love of learning. So what if I bombed early on? Even Julia Child acknowledged that it took her practice to learn a lot of things.

Cake 1 was a disaster, but I knew enough to laugh about it, and I wanted to improve. At cake 2, curiosity and love of learning kicked in: How will I know when the egg whites are just right? How do I know a flat cake tastes bad? By cake 3, I was onto the "folding process" (again, curiosity, love of learning, and I was still chuckling over my improving but less-than-perfect product). By cake 5, I was home free: perfection. I had achieved AFCSE— and not only that, AFCSE generalized to cheese soufflés.

Self-efficacy is an important ingredient of resilience, as well as an essential quality in developing into an authoritative (not authoritarian) parent for one's children. Like many other personal qualities and skills, it is particularly useful in parenting children at risk for disabilities and in living with family members who have incurred disabilities. Not only is self-efficacy developed in small steps, but it probably starts in self-recognition of mastering a few simple small things, like baking an angel food cake. Box 8–5 is a useful exercise for kick-starting self-efficacy and mastery.

After group members complete the exercise, discussion can focus on the following points:

- For parents, are there some important implications for role modeling self-trust for the family?
- Is it likely that your children will also benefit from developing self-trust? How can you help them to develop it?
- For families, how might your self-efficacy improve the situation for your disabled partner?
- How might you help your spouse to gain or regain some mastery?

### Activity Three: Reaching Out

Resilience is not a matter of taking what comes one's way, toughing it out, being the master of one's fate. Resilience is defined at some length in Chapter 2, but it also can be thought of simply as the "capacity to maintain competent function in the face of major life stressors" (Masten, Best, & Garmezy, 1990). Resilience involves many skills, as suggested previously, and reaching out is a critical one, both to check on one's perceptions and to position oneself to receive help from others. Reaching out, of course, also involves

---

**Box 8–5. Week 2: Trusting Yourself Exercise—
Parent and Family Version**

Each of us recognizes our mastery of something, however small. This *self-efficacy* serves to put us on the path to trust ourselves to handle bigger things. Describe one thing you can count on yourself to do well. How did you apply the three principles of practice, small steps, and applying one or more of your strengths?

*Parent version:*

Think of some aspect of your child raising to which you could apply these principles. Find a way to use the steps to teach your child a task that he or she can perform with confidence.

*Family version:*

Think of a small task, not necessarily communication related, that your spouse may be able to do successfully (or resume the responsibility for, e.g., separating coins by size and putting them in a coin dispenser, feeding the fish, balancing the checkbook). Help him or her to follow the three principles of practice, small steps, and applying a strength to do or resume doing the task.

---

being able to accept the reaching out of others, of learning to be honored and empowered by it. Box 8–6 contains an exercise that is designed as a first step to reaching out.

This is the final exercise for this session. Typically, everyone finds someone to reach out to, but the group leader may need to broker this process, either by getting some of the "strays" together or by personally reaching out to anyone who has not yet made contact with another participant. The exercise should take no more than 10 minutes or so. This is a "feel good" interaction for everyone, and one that provides an easy transition to discussion. Appropriate discussion questions include the following:

- Is there a balance between reaching out and going it alone?
- Can reaching out be giving as well as seeking?

> ### Box 8–6. Week 2: Reaching Out Exercise
>
> By now, you probably have noticed one person (at least) in the workshop whose comments have moved or impressed you, and whom you would like to get to know a little better. Or perhaps you have been touched by someone's problems and wish to find out more, if only to help a bit. Or perhaps you have been concerned about a person in the room who has been very shy and has difficulty speaking. Now reach out to that person in keeping with the basis for your interest —explore or share an insight, give a hug or a pat on the back, or encourage with supportive words.

- Reaching out also means finding support groups and websites. Does anyone have some they particularly wish to share? (The group leader may wish to make available as a handout a list of some of the websites from previous chapters that may be helpful.)

### Homework: Three Good Things Exercise

Box 8–7 presents another version of the "Three Good Things" exercise described in Chapter 2. It is particularly appropriate here because it combines aspects of self-efficacy in understanding the role an individual plays in causing positive emotions; reaching out, by recognizing others' roles. As before, the leader's role is to explain the exercise and encourage participants to write up their experiences in terms of what they have learned from it.

# Week 3

The major focus of Week 3 is on how to develop "optimistic explanatory style" (Peterson, 2006; Reivich & Shatté, 2002), part of the fabric of positive psychology. We are going to call this the ABCD approach, after Reivich and Shatté. Explanatory style in its essence

---

**Box 8–7. Week 2: Homework—Three Good Things**

*Parent version:*

- Begin each day this week by selecting a member of your family (spouse, child, yourself). Find a way to keep track, either by observation or asking, of three good things that happened to the chosen person each day. What did the person do to bring them about?
- Share this information with the chosen person at the end of the day.

*Family version:*

- For 3 days this week, focus on your family member. Either by observing or asking, find three good things that happened to him or her on those days. Before you go to bed, share your thoughts on what he or she did to bring them about.
- For 3 other days, focus on yourself. At the end of the day, summarize them to yourself, and determine what you did to bring them about.
- For the final day, turn the tables. Observe one good thing that happened to you today that came about because of something your family member did. Also, observe one good thing that happened to him or her because of something *you* did. Share the information before going to bed.

---

involves the perceptions and understandings people use in explaining events to themselves, how those explanations influence their behavior, and how they can, with practice, learn to recognize and change them, and as a result think more optimistically. The exercises that preceded Week 3 all have contributed to the process of improved self-awareness. But because explanatory style is not particularly transparent, but often hidden deep in personal belief systems and characteristic responses, this component of positive psychology is addressed directly here, along with finding some ways to challenge underlying beliefs. Communication counselors are urged to revisit Chapter 2 and also to explore Reivich and Shatté (2002) once again, to broaden their understanding of explanatory style beyond the simple introduction provided here.

Week 3 begins with a short lecture highlighting the following main points: When bad things happen to people, particularly events out of their control, they frequently experience feelings of helplessness. Having a child with a handicap can be such a situation, and as parents struggle to understand and to move with it, they attempt to understand why it has happened. This also is the situation for families when a family member experiences a catastrophic medical event. These are major adversities, but in daily life, many smaller but nevertheless upsetting adversities occur as well.

What each person brings to adversity (major or minor) is explanatory style—how that person explains adversity to himself or herself. Explanatory style tends to emerge from three sources: (1) internal factors versus external factors; (2) factors of permanence versus change; and (3) global factors versus local factors. Reivich and Shatté (2002) summarize these three factors as "me versus not me," "always versus sometimes," and "everything versus not everything," respectively. Each is briefly described next.

*Me versus not me* sets the locus of responsibility: "I am totally responsible for all that happens—good and bad—not only to me but also to those around me, and possibly in extreme cases, for everything that happens in my world." People with this outlook see themselves as those who bring these events about. For example, a "me" person may state: "It is my fault that Gustav had his stroke, because I didn't insist that he take it easy. He was working too hard, and I knew it." Conversely, a "not me" person takes little responsibility for what happens to him or her or their immediate others. It is the fault of someone or something else.

*Always versus seldom* sets the temporal locus. For example, someone at the extremes sees all events as unique at one pole or the way things always are—good and bad—at the other. Use of the words "never" and "always" is a good indicator of this style. Statements such as "Nothing like this illness has ever happened before to us" and "Illness and pain have always been a part of my experience" also provide some clues to this explanatory style.

Finally, there is the durability, or generalization, of *everything versus not everything*—the notion of "the way it always is" versus "unique to this one event." "This is the story of my life" implies "everything." "Nothing in my life prepared me for this" implies "not everything." All three factors are end points on a range; few people are at the extremes. In adversity-laden situations, however, people who are "addicted" to pessimism crowd around the *me, always, everything* end of the range, whereas "cockeyed optimists" are at the other end. The first exercise related to these continua appears in Box 8–8.

The goal is to help workshop participants situate themselves along each of the three continua, and to discuss how these reactions fuel their beliefs. Provide paper and use the examples in Box 8–8 to have participants rate themselves on the three dimensions.

After the rating has been completed, the discussion should focus on points such as the following:

- How beliefs influence behavior in relation to adversity . Use the example situations as stimuli for generating alternative actions. Refer to Box 8–4, which presents an exercise on recognizing feelings.
- How we can generate alternatives to them, again referring to the feelings exercise.
- The danger of extremes at each end of the continuum.

An important implication of this kind of analysis is how we explain the relationship between adversities, beliefs, and consequences, and how we can learn to change our behavior in relation to them. (A) stands for the adversities, (B) represents our beliefs in relationship to them, and (C) stands for the negative emotional consequences of those beliefs. Reivich and Shatté (2002) lay out a potent grid for examining the consequences of adversity, modulated by beliefs:

| **The Belief** | **Its Consequences** |
|---|---|
| Violation of one's rights | Anger |
| Real-world loss, or loss of self-worth | Sadness, depression |
| Violation of another's rights | Guilt |
| Future threat | Anxiety |
| Negative self-comparison with others | Embarrassment |

## Box 8–8. Week 3: "Me-Always-Everything" Examples of Explanatory Style for Adversities

*Parent version:*

*Adversity Example 1*

At the insistence of your family and your pediatrician, you made an appointment to have your child evaluated by the city's leading neuropsychologist. It took 6 months to get the appointment, and today is the big day, but your child woke up with a temperature of 103°, and you have to cancel the appointment. How could this have happened?

> *Belief:* I should have been very careful to keep him out of drafts and away from kids who were not well, so that he would have been shipshape today.

> Is this a good explanation for you? Rate it on the following scale:

> **This is totally due to me.    This is just circumstance.**
> 1    2    3    4    5    6    7

> *Belief:* It's probably silly to make another appointment, because it will just happen again.

> **Such stuff always happens.    It will not happen again.**
> 1    2    3    4    5    6    7

> *Belief:* That's the way life is. I can't win.

> **It is the story of my life.    It is a unique circumstance.**
> 1    2    3    4    5    6    7

*Adversity Example 2*

You had a really hard day at work, and when you got home, you discovered that your 10-year-old had misplaced her house key, so she went to the neighbor's house, where she watched TV instead of doing her homework. She also could not do her chore for the day, which was to take dinner out of the freezer, and you have no backup supper dish. You threw a fit.

*Belief:* **I expect too much from my kids.**                    **It was all her fault.**

   1     2     3     4     5     6     7

*Belief:* **That is the way it is going to be.**               **It will never happen again.**

   1     2     3     4     5     6     7

*Belief:* **Everything goes this way.**                    **It is a unique event.**

   1     2     3     4     5     6     7

*Family version:*

*Adversity Example 1*

Since Hugh's stroke, you have had to go back to work, and be responsible for getting him to therapy, being sure he's picked up by the Handi-Car service at the right time, and brought home again every day. You ask your sister to check in to see that all is going according to schedule. You come home on Wednesday after a hard day, and Hugh is not there. The new Handi-Car driver forgot to pick him up and the speech clinic secretary calls to ask when you are going to pick him up.

*Belief:* **This is my fault— I should have reminded my sister to remind the driver.**            **My sister is a ditz brain.**

   1     2     3     4     5     6     7

*Belief:* **It is always this way—nothing goes right.**            **All will be well when the new driver learns the ropes.**

   1     2     3     4     5     6     7

*Belief:* **This stroke is ruining our whole life.**            **Some snafus are bound to occur.**

   1     2     3     4     5     6     7

*Adversity Example 2*

Your neighbor calls to tell you that your wife, Alice, who has mild dementia, is walking alone down the street in her nightgown, asking everyone the way to the church you both used to attend, and that it is Sunday and she is late for services (it is Wednesday).

| *Belief:* **It is all my fault—How did I not notice she'd left?** | | | | | **Not my fault—she must have found the front door key.** | |
|---|---|---|---|---|---|---|
| 1 | 2 | 3 | 4 | 5 | 6 | 7 |

| *Belief:* **I have to keep an eye on her all the time.** | | | | | **A new lock will take care of it.** | |
|---|---|---|---|---|---|---|
| 1 | 2 | 3 | 4 | 5 | 6 | 7 |

| *Belief:* **Soon she will be wandering everywhere.** | | | | | **Church was so important to her—this was an isolated event.** | |
|---|---|---|---|---|---|---|
| 1 | 2 | 3 | 4 | 5 | 6 | 7 |

To learn to change one's responses to adversity, whether for parents dealing with the teacher who does not quite understand their concerns about their child or for a family member dealing with a doctor who cannot predict a time course for recovery from TBI, one has first to understand these connections. That's the ABCs of it. The next step is examining the connections, and to provide oneself with counter-arguments (disputing them is the D component of this approach) that encourage flexibility in problem solving and developing resilience. Now we have the ABCD of "hot seating" (Peterson, 2006) or of developing "real-time resilience" (Reivich & Shatté, 2002).

## Developing Alternative Ways of Thinking: The ABCD Approach

The second exercise, and a pivotal one, begins the process of confronting one's explanatory style. Essentially, the approach involves learning to: (1) evaluate the evidence for one's immediate response, (2) think of alternative ways of explaining the situation, and (3) use these alternatives as the basis for developing a different approach to the adversity. The crucial questions are as follows:

- What alternatives are available as explanations?
- Can I practice arguing with my initial reaction? Can I come up with alternative explanations?
- What difference would it make? Is there value in changing my response?
- How can I apply this to my life?

Peterson (2006) suggests using another trusted person, aware of the process, to provide counterpoint and aid in developing alternatives. Although practicing with another person may be necessary for some persons early on, once they have identified their own explanatory style, and have practiced often enough, most people can (and in the long run should) serve this function for themselves.[5]

Box 8–9 presents two extended examples, one for parents of a child with moderate cerebral palsy and one for family members—in this case the spouse of an aphasic man. These examples provide problem-oriented material for discussion in their respective workshops. A useful follow-up exercise is to have workshop participants pair off and continue practice, as described in Box 8–10.

The session ends with an exercise based on the gratitude visit, one of the most moving of the exercises for which Seligman, Steen, Park, and Peterson (2005) have provided efficacy data. This exercise was introduced in Chapter 2. It is simply the act of remembering someone to whom you are especially grateful, and whom you have never properly thanked for whatever this person has done for you. Once you have chosen your recipient, write a short (i.e., one page or so) letter of gratitude; then schedule a meeting or a phone call and simply read the letter aloud to the person being thanked. Then evaluate the effects not only on the person but also on yourself.

---

[5]From a personal perspective, Audrey learned and then practiced "real-time resilience." Although it took a lot of careful practice early on, I can attest that it became easier and is now almost automatic. One of its joys is that mental "hot seating" is serviceable for concerns as diverse as why I have had an unsatisfactory interaction with a coaching client and why my garbage disposal once again is giving me fits.

**Box 8–9. Week 3: Problem-Oriented Issues for Illustrating ABCD—Family and Parent Version**

*Example 1* "Real-Time Resilience": Adults

The following resilience approach for aphasic adults is based on Reivich and Shatté's (2002) ABCD approach.

The problem: "I can't leave him alone. What if he had another stroke?"

The goal: Dissect into adversity (A), beliefs (B), and consequences (C); then dispute them (D).

The view of the spouse, Jennifer:

A = ADVERSITY: George had a stroke and cannot talk.

B = BELIEF: I cannot leave him alone, because what if he had another stroke?

*Uncovered thinking trap* and connection between beliefs and consequences: If he has another stroke, and I am not there to get help, I am afraid he will die. I will be responsible for his death.

C = CONSEQUENCES

*Emotional consequences:* I feel anxious. I will be responsible for his death. I am angry. I have to take George everywhere I go.

*Behavioral consequences:* That is no fun for either of us. I am trapped. I do not have any time to myself.

D = DISPUTATION: Let us think this through:

- Is this realistic? What are the odds?
- Do we have any safeguards in place in case he needs help? (e.g., augmentative devices, medical alert system, panic button on house alarm). The answer is yes to all of these.
- Does Jennifer have any backup alternatives? Friends, children, help in the house who could give her free time? The answer is yes.
- Does Jennifer know how George views this state of affairs? The answer is no.

The view of George, the severely aphasic spouse:

A = ADVERSITY: Jennifer will not leave me alone since the stroke.

B = BELIEF: She thinks I am incompetent.

*Uncovered thinking trap:* If my wife of 30 years thinks I am incompetent, I must be.

C = CONSEQUENCES

*Emotional consequences:* I am angry with Jennifer for not believing in me. I am frustrated because I have no choices. I am sad because she thinks I am incompetent.

*Behavioral consequences:* I have to go everywhere that Jennifer goes. I feel trapped. I do not have any time to myself.

D = DISPUTATION

Because George is severely aphasic, probably the foregoing intact internal dialogue cannot be expressed, or will be expressed in emotional ways (registering anger, frustration, and sadness); therefore, the disputation is largely in Jennifer's terms. Each of her points can be disputed, as follows: Does George's anger and frustration make sense? Yes, it does. Jennifer's behavior belies his cognitive competence. Another stroke is possible, certainly, but regular doctor visits are in place, medications are taken systematically, and he does not need constant supervision during speech therapy. Furthermore, nobody checks on his opinion.

- Is George incompetent? No, he just cannot talk.
- Are there safeguards? George has a backup, simple augmentative system for calling 911 and also has a medical alert system in place.
- Family and friends have offered to stay with George but have never been called to do so.
- Because it is not easy to get George's side in the disputation, a clinician may play George's part, as described. George ideally is present for this and is encouraged to agree or disagree.

Develop a plan of action with three steps:

1. Validate George's point of view.
2. Use appropriate questions, or have a clinician role-play George's part, as described previously. George is present and encouraged to agree or disagree.
3. Test the realities uncovered in the disputation:

   ■ Call in the daughter-in-law to stay with George while Jennifer goes to the beauty shop. Did George have a stroke? Repeat as necessary to collect data. Then try successive trips away alone (e.g., take a 5-minute walk, go to the Starbuck's on the corner and bring George a cup of his favorite coffee, go for a 15-minute walk). Collect the data. Evaluate everyone's feelings.

   ■ Help Jennifer to learn the technique so that she can do it on her own for other situations. You may wish to use the technique yourself to address one of your own problems. Experience using it helps you to explain it.

*Example 2* "Real-Time Resilience": Children

The following resilience approach developed for the parents of Halston, a 6-year-old boy with moderate-severe cerebral palsy including dysarthria, is based on Reivich and Shatté's (2002) ABCD approach.

The problem: The school wants to mainstream Halston for first grade.

The goal: Dissect into adversity (A), beliefs (B), and consequences (C); then dispute them (D).

The view of the parents, Ada and Clark:

A = ADVERSITY: His schoolmates will not accept Halston.

B = BELIEFS: Halston needs to be protected. He does not understand. We, not the school, should be making this decision.

*Uncovered thinking traps* and connections between beliefs and consequences: We have invested great energy in making his world safe. This investment will be lost. Underneath it all, we have doubts about Halston's abilities. Our rights are being violated.

C = CONSEQUENCES

*Emotional consequences:* We feel anxious. We feel angry. We are embarrassed.

*Behavioral consequences:* We are confronting the school.

D = DISPUTATION: Let us think this through.

- Is this realistic? What are the odds?
- The school has tested Halston. They feel he is fine.
- Has Halston been okay in his interactions with other children? The answer is yes.
- Are there other things as important as being protected? The answer is yes. Such things include acceptance by others, which cannot happen without trying.
- Is there help available for Halston and us? Yes.

Develop a plan of action with two steps:

1. Test the realities uncovered in the disputation.
   - Before school starts, invite some of his potential classmates over to play. See what happens. Get the data.
   - Check with your older children.
   - Talk to the school about your concerns; gain assurance of their help. Develop an acceptable alternative plan together with the school.
   - Find out what Halston thinks about going to first grade.

2. Help Ada and Clark learn the technique so that they can use it in other situations. You may wish to use the technique yourself to address one of your own problems. Experience using it helps you to explain it.

*Note*: This adversity has been less fully described than that involving George and Jennifer, primarily because the model is transparent enough to permit easy elaboration. Notice that this one has many possible permutations. For example, what if Ada and Clark differed in their opinions about whether or not to mainstream Halston? What about Halston's own opinions, and those of his siblings?

---

**Box 8–10. Week 3: Pair-off Practice with
"Real-Time Resilience"**

Any of the scenarios described in Box 8–4 or Box 8–8 can
serve as adversity examples (or, for that matter, many of the
"counseling moments"). This pairing-off exercise concerns
what beliefs are triggered by the adversity and the consequences that follow. One participant takes the role of the
person who has had the adversity; the other, the role of the
colleague who helps figure out alternatives to the beliefs.
When the necessary goals have been achieved for the selected
adversity example, the participants switch roles. It also is possible, even preferable, for people to describe and to work
through their own adversities. Group leaders are encouraged
to be as creative as possible in developing scenarios. By now,
the workshop participants have become pretty well known to
each other, and appropriate scenarios can be developed for
specific pairings of participants.

---

The gratitude visit becomes the first assignment of the week,
that is, to plan and carry out a gratitude visit. The second assignment is to apply "real-time resilience" in a few instances that arise
during the week. Both of these assignments should be recorded in
the notebook or on evaluation sheets.

## Week 4: Wrap-Up

Week 4 is intended to be an uplifting and very pleasant, informal
experience. The goal is to launch participants into further explorations in the arena of living as fully and authentically as possible,
and to support their continued use of the kinds of resilience-build-
ing activities that are the focus of the workshop. The first activity of
the week, therefore, is to share the experiences the group has had
in planning and carrying out their gratitude visits. This usually is a
momentous and significant activity for most members of the group,
who seem at first surprised to find that they have gotten perhaps

even more than they have given as they planned and carried out the exercise. Discussion points are many and varied and include at least the following:

- Can you consider making other gratitude visits? For example, is there someone who has been particularly helpful to you in dealing with your child or your spouse? What about thanking some members of your own family?
- Gratitude visits often are costly in terms of planning and execution. What are other, simpler ways to similar (if less dramatic) ends?
- Why is expressing gratitude so powerful?

Experiences in changing explanatory style through real-time resilience and hot seating also should be examined. These experiences can initiate a general discussion of what individuals have learned or achieved from the workshop, and how future workshops can be improved. The facilitator may wish to provide handouts that will help people continue to apply what they have learned in the workshop. Many additional exercises can be found throughout this book. The suggestions inspired by Masten and Reed (2005), and presented in Box 8–11, can be used as an effective handout for parents.

It is important at the last session to leave enough time for interpersonal networking and visiting, and it is our preference to conclude with refreshments and enough time to tie up loose ends informally. Workshops invariably provide an intense learning experience for both facilitators and participants; therefore, the group leader may wish to conclude with his or her own gratitude statement to the participants.

## Variations on the Workshop Theme

### Adolescents with Communication Disorders

The format for this workshop variant remains the same. The exercises, from the parents and family versions, can easily be adapted for use with adolescents with communication disorders, or for that

---

**Box 8–11. Week 4: Strategies for Promoting Resilience in Children with Disabilities**

■ Build self-efficacy through small steps; practice simple things first.
■ Teach coping strategies for specific situations.
■ Foster secure attachment relationships between you and your child.
■ Seek help from other families and other experts.
■ Participate in programs designed for special needs for children in your community.
■ Seek trustworthy support from Internet resources.
■ Help your child to establish friendships with other children.
■ Support cultural traditions that provide children with adaptive rituals and opportunities to bond with other children and adults (e.g., religious education, Little League, Special Olympics).

---

(Inspired by Masten and Reed, 2005.)

---

matter, with any child who has the appropriate maturity. In addition to these exercises, the exercises that conclude Chapter 5, almost without exception, can be fitted into the framework of this workshop. For example, exercises 8, 9, and 10 are all versions of the gratitude visit; the mishap scenarios from the laugh-lesson exercise can be used for real-time resilience; exercises 4 and 7 both fit well into the theme of building trust in oneself. Possibly the biggest difference from the more standard format is that communication counselors should be especially alert to fostering strong peer relationships among participants throughout the workshop. Because these focused workshops are likely to be small, this should not be difficult. It also usually is possible to pay closer attention to individual participants' needs. Because, as previously discussed, there is some emerging evidence of the effectiveness of cognitive-behavioral therapy (CBT) in the management of some communication disorders, one goal of this workshop, in addition to the general goals discussed previously, may be to encourage some group members to participate in CBT.

## Adults with Aphasia

Again, the explicit format of the workshop experience for adults with aphasia should not differ markedly in terms of either the topics covered or the types of exercises undertaken. The family variant, rather than the parent variant, is used. Once again, counselors are encouraged to revisit previous chapters for appropriate exercises that have been especially adapted for persons with aphasia.

Although the format may not vary significantly, implementation for adults with aphasia requires some modifications. First, it probably is not possible to do all of the exercises and discuss them fully in the constrained time frame, unless participation is limited to persons with mild aphasia. Because people with more moderate problems, and even some with severe aphasias, can profit from this experience, one solution is to use fewer exercises.

Another variation may be to double the number of sessions, but it seems more appropriate simply to repeat the experience for those who are interested, and change the exercises in the second series. Another recommended modification is to limit group size to 10 to 12 participants, to ensure balanced participation. Finally, this workshop variation must include "supported communication" procedures, and to ensure implementation of this support, at least two group leaders are necessary.

## Adults with Hearing Loss

With adults who have incurred hearing loss, there is a need not only to teach them about unfamiliar technologies, such as cochlear implants, assistive devices, and hearing aids, but also about how to use them appropriately. It is also necessary to instruct them in how to modify their attitudes, beliefs, and listening strategies, as well as to help close others to learn relevant new skills. In effect, it is not enough to provide a hearing aid or listening device and an hour of instruction. One comprehensive group program geared to teaching both management of hearing loss, and living well with it, is currently ongoing at the University of Arizona. Three weeks in length, this program meets once weekly for two hours per week with individuals who have hearing loss and their significant others. Although the words "positive psychology" are probably never mentioned, this workshop meets and achieves the same sorts of goals we have laid out for other problems in this chapter. For a detailed description of the program and its validation, see Marrone and Harris (2012).

## Conclusion

This chapter does not present an experimental protocol or a series of lesson plans, but rather a set of guidelines for creating meaningful workshop experiences for adults and children who have communication disorders, and for their significant others. Nevertheless, clinicians interested in conducting such a workshop are urged to collect as much information as possible concerning its utility. Both qualitative and quantitative data are appropriate. Workshops such as these are perhaps the most significant departures from traditional approaches to the management of speech, language, and hearing disorders that are discussed in this book, yet they have potential for increasing the quality of life for the clients we serve. If they are to be viable, supporting documentation is mandatory.

## References

Heath, C., & Heath, D. (2010). *Switch: How to change things when change is hard*. New York, NY: Broadway Books.

Marrone, N., & Harris, F. (2012). A multifaceted living well approach to the management of hearing loss with adults and their frequent communication partners. *Perspectives on Aural Rehabilitation and Its Instrumentation, 19*(1), 5–14.

Masten, A. S., Best, K. M., & Garmezy, N. (1990). Resilience and development: Contributions from the study of children who overcome adversity. *Development and Psychopathology, 2*, 425–444.

Masten, A. S., & Reed, M. G. (2005). Resilience in development. In C. Snyder & S. Lopez (Eds.), *Handbook of positive psychology*. Oxford, UK: Oxford University Press.

Peterson, C. (2006). *A primer in positive psychology*. New York, NY: Oxford University Press.

Reivich, K., & Shatté, A. (2002). *The resilience factor: Seven essential skills for overcoming life's inevitable obstacles.* New York, NY: Broadway Books.

Seligman, M. (2002). *Authentic happiness.* New York, NY: Free Press.

Seligman, M. (2011). *Flourish.* New York, NY: Free Press

Seligman, M. E. P., Steen, T. A., Park, N., & Peterson, C. (2005). Positive psychology progress: Empirical validation of interventions. *American Psychologist, 60*(5), 410–421.

# Chapter 9

# THERE'S AN ELEPHANT IN THE ROOM: ISSUES IN DEATH AND DYING

## Stan Goldberg

## Foreword

It seems totally fitting that this book on counseling across the life-span should conclude with a chapter on end-of-life issues dealt with positively and directly. Today's clinicians who work in extended care facilities increasingly encounter clients who are dying, but little in their coursework has prepared them for the experience of the death of a person with whom they have formed a rather intimate association. In my own counseling courses, I have relied on Stan Goldberg, who once was my student and now is my teacher in this and many other topics, to guide me. His experiences as a hospice worker and as a gifted communication counselor and clinician make him a uniquely qualified authority on the issues of death and dying in communication counseling. Initially I had asked him only for help with this chapter; when later he graciously volunteered to write it himself, I accepted it as the gift of loving-kindness that it is. Read it with care and respect.

—Audrey L. Holland

## Introduction

Death is like the strange relative we speak about in whispers, and then only when children are not present. Even though we try to keep death from conscious thought, discomfort bubbles up when we encounter a patient who is obviously dying. We tell her how good she looks despite her sunken cheeks and sallow complexion. We are tongue-tied—not because we do not care, but because we fear death.

Those of us who are courageous enough to hold the gaze may read books such as Elisabeth Kübler-Ross's *On Death and Dying* (Kübler-Ross, 1997). In it and others equally insightful, the process of dying is calmly and objectively explained. But as the linguist Korzybski (1958) said, "The map is not the territory." Death cannot be known through dispassionate reading. Neither is it grasped by discussing "management" issues such as hospital rules, universal precautions, Medicare billing policies, demographics, or practices based on the American Speech-Language-Hearing Association's (ASHA) code of ethics. No, the experience of death is personal—an event so rich that just like a gourmet dish, it cannot be adequately described through words (Goldberg, 2009a); thus, I do not try to do so in this chapter. Instead, the chapter explores events and emotional states that surround death, and how you can have a significant impact on the quality of your patient's life, whether it is measured in months or even hours (Goldberg, 2010a, 2012).

There is a Tibetan saying that to get over those things that are feared the most, draw them in close (Patrul Rinpoche, 1994). How to get "chummy" with death is the theme of this chapter, which looks at what communication counselors can contribute to dying patients, and what you, as a human being, can learn from the experience.

# Why Practice Speech or Language Therapy with the Dying?

I remember a conversation I had with my mother when I decided to become a speech-language pathologist (SLP). She was a wonderful but simple woman. As she got older, there were things she had more difficulty understanding than her friends did about their children—like my choice of profession. "Speech-language pathology?" she asked. "What's that?" After carefully explaining what I did, I thought she understood until I heard her talking to a friend: "He's a speech-language pathologist. You know, someone who helps children move their tongues." No, she did not get it right 30 years ago. But as I look at ASHA's current scope of practice for SLPs, I find her description prophetic. We have moved in the direction of being highly competent specialists—technically more precise, but now maybe less willing to go beyond moving tongues (Goldberg, 2003).

## Scope of Practice

We have strayed from the first visions our profession's founders had more than 70 years ago. Although they wanted us to correct speech and language problems, they also believed we had another obligation to our clients. They viewed the people they served as whole human beings who needed not only technical services but also compassion. (Therapy for the dying is not about technical competency—*it is about facilitating painful communications.*)

When people near their own death, suppressed emotions and fears surface as if the barriers confining them had become porous. As a hospice volunteer, I was with a woman in her nineties who vividly remembered the beatings her mother gave her when she was 5 years of age. She repeated the story to each person caring for her in a hospice facility, even acting it out when morphine made her delirious. Although I was there as a bedside volunteer, my training and experience as a speech-language pathologist enabled me to help her communicate her pain, not only to others but also to herself.

## Competency in Communication

As professionals, we have become prisoners of our name. Years ago, we were "speech pathologists." As the importance of differentiating between language and speech problems gained momentum, we became "speech-language pathologists." Now, we call ourselves "aphasiologists," or "early language interventionists," or "speech-language pathologists with an emphasis in _____" (fill in the blank). The increasing narrowing of how we identify ourselves reflects a changing focus on what we do, or are willing to do.

We focus on correcting specific speech and language disorders as if that were the final goal—but it is not. Speech and language are just *tools* of communication. We work on helping our clients develop and use these tools to facilitate communication. When we dwell less on our newly acquired parochialism, our competency in correcting specific disorders becomes the means for achieving a greater goal. We become *communication counselors*, who also are competent to work on helping clients develop and use their tools for communicating.

## Painful Communications: What Are They?

A number of years ago at a workshop, Sogyal Rinpoche (1993) related a conversation a counselor had with a dying patient. The patient said he did not need to have anyone understand what he was going through; that was not possible. Rather, he just wanted people to *act* as if they did. I do not claim special knowledge when it comes to death, although I have taken the journey often with others. Like everyone else, I have to wait until it is my turn to know what death is about. But as a hospice volunteer, I have seen reoccurring communication problems emanating from the impending experience of death in both children and adults. It is possible to do more than just act as if we understand what our patient is experiencing (Goldberg, 2010b).

The initial step is understanding that the dying process is physically and psychologically messy. By its very nature, it continually changes, moving persons through the most dramatic changes they will experience (Goldberg, 2006). Change is difficult for most people to accept, even under ordinary circumstances. When change occurs gradually, it can be made more acceptable (Goldberg, 1997). But with terminal illnesses, change occurs as if it sits on an out-of-control conveyer belt, ignoring the wishes of the person whose life it is changing.

With lingering terminal illnesses, personalities change by necessity—rarely by choice. One's place within their world changes as patients are forced to move from independence to dependence, health to illness, and being in control to having none at all. The difficulties they encounter often become apparent when they try to communicate their psychological pain. Four recurring themes are adjusting to changes, expressing gratitude, regrets, and the need to simplify. Within each of these areas of concern, communication counselors have the knowledge to alleviate suffering.

## The Unsettling Nature of Change

For the person who is dying, a world that may have been as solid as concrete becomes as unstable as a bowl of Jell-O. Tibetans have a word for this rootless psychological state. They call it the *bardo* (Sogyal Rinpoche, 1994). Although the term is traditionally reserved for the time between death and the consciousness leaving the body, it can be applied to transitions from who a person was to who that person is becoming (Goldberg, 2002). There is discomfort in transitions, sometimes even fear. People are moving from something they know to an unknown. Some people believe the fear of death may have more to do with giving up what is familiar than dreading what happens after their last breath (Krishnamurti, 1994).

I have witnessed family members and friends unable to understand such changes. Knowing the person was dying, they still expected that person to act the same as before becoming ill. When the kind, happy, accepting person becomes belligerent and is no longer interested in anything but his or her own memories, support from puzzled loved ones often vanishes. Communication counselors can enable the person who is dying to express the fears he or she may be feeling, and if not, at least convey to loved ones why the changes are occurring.

### What to Do

- Expect your patients to have sudden mood shifts.
- Do not minimize the changes they are experiencing.
- If patients ask what it is like to die, tell them—if you know. If you do not, find someone who has been with people who have died.
- Do not initiate discussions about dying. If and when patients are ready to talk about it, they will let you know.
- Accept every change in your patient's personality. Do not expect consistency.
- Help patients express the fear they are experiencing to friends and family.
- When patients cannot express their fear, you should convey it to family and friends.

## Gratitude: Giving and Receiving

Accepting gratitude can be a public statement of personal need. The grateful person who is dying may be saying "I can't do it anymore by myself." For people who have taken pride in being independent their entire lives, expressing gratitude may be difficult. Such difficulties also may signal a denial of their condition (Emmons, 2004).

Bruce, a retired educator, came to a hospice facility in San Francisco where I was a bedside volunteer. He had congestive heart failure and was obsessively independent. As he grew weaker, Irma, a very considerate staff person, tried to help him. He not only refused all of her efforts but often would yell at her. Allowing anyone to help meant he was dying, something he could not accept. Once, after being screamed at and cursed, Irma quietly said, "I know you don't want my help now, but I want you to know, when you can accept it, I'll be here for you."

For two weeks he refused all offers of help, causing himself needless pain. I was alone with him when he had to urinate and realized his urinal was full. With great hesitation, he apologetically asked me to empty it. When I returned, he spent the next 10 minutes repeatedly thanking me. The gratitude he expressed was totally out of proportion to what I thought I had done. I made the mistake of saying, "It was nothing." In my mind, what I did was routine. To Bruce, asking me to empty a urinal meant the acceptance of dependence and his terminal condition.

### What to Do

- When someone offers thanks, accept it without qualification.
- Understand that being grateful can be embarrassing.
- The smallest gesture of kindness to a person who is dying can have enormous consequences.

## Regrets

As people approach death, they often have regrets about things they did and things they wish they had done. Regrets often take the form of goals not achieved, apologies owed, and apologies needed. Professionals are inclined either to minimize these concerns or to switch the conversation to less painful topics. Unfortunately, these decisions often reflect their own level of comfort more than their patients' needs. Unless these difficult issues are resolved, they may become barriers to a more peaceful death.

## Unmet Goals

Western civilization is goal driven. We strive to achieve specific things: to amass money, to live comfortably, to become a successful SLP, and so forth. Our patients also are a product of the society in which they live (Weber, 1946). They are as logs floating down a river. Although each moves differently, all are being carried downstream by the flow of water. Patients whose lives have been goal directed often focus on things they have not achieved, regardless of their accomplishments. If they dwell on such things as they approach death, it is significant, even if, in the general scheme of life, it actually is not.

I cared for a well-known journalist who had written 10 books (as well as hundreds of newspaper columns during the Second World War) throughout his illustrious life. Many people believed he was responsible for changing how war stories were reported. His prostate cancer had metastasized, and approaching death, he fixated on an unfinished magazine article he knew would never be completed. Despite having accomplished more in his life than most other journalists, he could focus only on the incomplete article —one he acknowledged would be a "minor contribution." It can be difficult to console people who view their lives as a series of unfulfilled dreams.

## Apologies: To Be Given and Received

We all can identify things we are sorry we did, and for which we would like to receive forgiveness. We also have been on the receiving end of painful words and actions we vividly remember years after they occurred. As people approach death, wanting to be forgiven and wanting to forgive become important. For people who are runners, it is like a burr in your sock that prevents you from feeling good about your run, no matter how fast it was. Not forgiving or receiving forgiveness can prevent people from having a "good death" (Kapleau, 1989).

When I first met Ethel, an 82-year-old woman with pulmonary failure, her dementia was just beginning. During each of my first three weekly visits, she repeated a story of how she, as an elementary school teacher, was ignored by other teachers in her school. As she told and retold the detailed story, reliving the 40-year-old experience changed a beautiful smiling face into one clearly in pain. I spent many hours with her trying to explore how the other teachers' inadequacies may have caused them to do hurtful things. After 2 months of conversations, she was finally able to forgive their cruelty. It is moot whether they were justified in snubbing her. My concern was to do whatever was necessary to help her death be more peaceful than it would have been if she had continued to harbor 40-year-old resentments.

### What to Do

- Let patients express their regrets and acknowledge the importance of such expression to them.
- Help them examine the factors beyond their control that prevented them from achieving goals.
- Try to redirect the focus to things they achieved without minimizing what they did not achieve.

- If the patient needs to be forgiven by someone who is still alive, help him or her construct the dialog to express it. If those people are dead, or not available to receive the apology, ask the patient to dictate a letter to the person.
- If the patient wants to forgive someone, use the same procedures cited for being forgiven.
- Help the patient understand that often insensitivity is a reflection of one's own needs, rather than something negative about the unfortunate person at the receiving end of it.

## Simplification

One of the tenets of most Eastern religions and philosophies is the importance of simplifying life (Hanh, 2000). Although it is a choice for how we live, it becomes a necessity for most people who are dying. Life, for many, is analogous to a complicated musical piece, such as Mahler's "Fifth Symphony" or Billy Strayhorn's *"Take the A Train."* In both compositions it is possible to hear numerous instruments, the melody, the chord changes, the variations, and so forth. But to understand the piece, it must be reduced to the basic melody. For people who are dying, it is the melody of their lives they strive to hear. It is accomplished through a stripping-away process wherein most unimportant things are disregarded.

This is true for adults and children, although the stripping away is expressed differently in each age group. For example, with children, safety comes from being quietly held by an adult, rather than playing with their familiar toys. Adults give up pretenses and ignore social niceties, and as egos dissolve, role-related behaviors stop. At all ages, verbal communication dwindles. Unfortunately, many people misinterpret this as "withdrawal." The stripping-away process can take many forms. Sometimes it is subtle, as when a person who was on top of current events no longer cares to read a newspaper. Other times it is more blatant, as when a well-known poet decided to give herself a going-away party. She invited friends to her hospice facility, and after everyone told her how she had changed their lives, she called each person individually to her side. In a whisper, she said something and then gave each person a single sheet of paper on which one of her poems was written. When all of her poems were given away, she turned calmly to everyone and softly said, "Now, I'm ready to die." Few simplification processes are as dramatic as that one, but you will see it happen with everyone. It is almost as if the person is preparing for a trip to a foreign country and is limited to carrying 50 pounds of baggage. What is this person going to take? This choice, for your patients, will determine how they die. I was with a woman who was actively dying and talked about terrible things in her life. She was agitated and frightened. I reminded her of the intense love she felt for her granddaughter, and helped her to simplify her thoughts by eliminating everything except the image of her granddaughter cuddled next to her in bed.

### What to Do

- Understand that past interests may fade away as the person approaches death.
- Recognize that interests will become basic: Are people listening to me? Do people love me? What do I need for this journey?
- Help patients focus on the most important things that give them peace.

## Techniques for Facilitating Painful Communication

Communication is multidimensional. We do it through our thoughts, words, touch, presence, and even silence. If done correctly, it can heal the soul of the person who is dying and give comfort to family and friends.

### Listen

The need to listen can be placed on a long continuum. At one end are people who believe there is little or nothing to be learned from their students. At the other end are people who view everything in life as a source of knowledge. Probably at no time in our experience as communication counselors is it more important to recognize the knowledge inherent (the expertise) in those in whom we counsel.

Most people who are dying, whether an 85-year-old with metastasized cancer or a 6-year-old with cystic fibrosis, are in greater need of someone willing to listen than they are of someone ready to act or solve problems on their behalf (Goldberg, 2005a). It has been noted many times in this book that one of the hardest things for us to do as professionals is listen without judging. It is essential to understand that our patients know more about their needs and condition than we do (Goldberg, 1997), and if we just listen, we may become as knowledgeable as they are.

Many people believe that as someone approaches death, the person's need to communicate diminishes. Actually, the reverse is true. Unfortunately, we misperceive a reduction in words as a reduction in need. People who are dying are facing the most profound transition of their lives. Everything about them is changing. Silence in the dying may signal great uncertainty or fear, not the desire to be uncommunicative. Sogyal Rinpoche has said that speaking is for entertainment, but silence is for great wisdom (1994).

Listening is curative to the person who is being listened to and the one listening. Most people who are dying desperately want to talk about their lives and their deaths with someone who will silently, nonjudgmentally listen. As a hospice volunteer, I have often listened to people coming to terms with the end of their life: an 86-year-old who reviewed a life of blessings; a teenager whose only regret was the emotional pain he was causing his mother; a child realizing she will never become a ballerina. I have also listened to the last breaths of a woman as I silently held her hand and felt the pain she experienced living on the street her entire adult life. The most profound communication came from a dying infant I held in my arms as her life refused to leave. Listening is more than not talking. It becomes the ability to be in tune with a person's needs, whether it is breathing in unison or holding the hand of someone struggling with pain that cannot be dulled by morphine.

We are uncomfortable with silence, often filling it with word-fluff that does little more than mark time until something of significance can be said. As professionals, we need to resist this temptation.

### What to Do

- When you are with a dying person, sit closely with the chair facing the bed.
- Do not assume that silence means there is no desire to communicate.

- Silence is a form of communication.
- Simplify emotionally difficult concepts.
- Allow your patient to choose the discussion topics.

## Using Healing Communications

People who are dying often have a heightened sense of awareness —they are looking for anything that will help them understand their lives and accept their deaths (Goldberg, 2009b). Assume everything you say has importance. That does not mean you need to fret over every word; rather, if you understand your role, needless verbiage is naturally reduced. It is also useful to think about words as only one way of communicating. You can "talk" by touch, nonverbal behaviors, playing a soothing instrument, such as a Native American flute, and just being present. When I am with patients, "words" are the least desirable method of developing a bond. If I can convey a feeling through any other means of communication, I do.

I was asked to visit a homeless schizophrenic who was dying of lung cancer at a hospice facility. During my first visit, he did not say more than 20 words. As I sat next to him, he would occasionally glance at me and then quickly avert his eyes. After nearly an hour of silence, I said, "I have to go now. Thank you for letting me visit with you. Would you like me to return next week?" I expected him to remain silent or say "no." Instead, without any hesitation and while looking directly at me, he said, "Yes, I'd like that a lot." Our second meeting began as the first did. Then, after about 15 minutes of silence, he said, "I'm afraid of dying. Do you know what it's like?" I told him what I had experienced with the deaths of other people. We talked for over half an hour, with him initiating the topics that concerned him. My role was to help him formulate into words those things that previously were too frightening to talk or even think about.

### What to Do

- Do not rush to fill the silence.
- Touch, if the patient feels comfortable with it.
- Listen more, talk less. Think about listening 80% of the time.
- Keep noise to a minimum.

## Witnessing

"Witnessing" is not used here in a religious sense. It simply means acknowledging the person's condition and what they are experiencing. Witnessing a person's terminal illness, nonjudgmentally, can be one of the greatest gifts you can give—not just as a communication counselor but also as a caring person. It requires compassion: the ability to place oneself in another's shoes. It may be difficult to feel compassion for people who brought on their own demise, such as a lifelong smoker, a drug addict, or someone who practiced unsafe sex. Thich Nhat Hanh, the Vietnamese Buddhist monk, thought it was possible to feel compassion for anyone by visualizing the person as one's mother (Hanh, 1991). After all, how could you deny love to someone who nurtured you when you were helpless?

I found the visualization useful when I cared for Bill, a man who was dying of hepatitis. Every Friday we would drive to Lands End, a scenic place in San Francisco, and watch the Golden Gate Bridge to our right and the Pacific Ocean to our left. As Bill smoked his medical marijuana to stop the nausea from his pain medication, he talked about his life. As much as I wanted to probe, it was important for him to tell someone his life story, without being judged. So I rarely asked questions, and when I did, it was for clarification. Although his lifestyle and some of his values were different from mine, I was there not to judge but to allow him to communicate. At one of our last outings, he told me of events in his life he had never shared with anyone. When he finished, he looked more peaceful than he ever had before. He said he felt comfortable telling me because he needed to talk about these life events without being judged.

### *What to Do*

- Do not impose your needs or understanding of how the world should be.
- Accept your patient's perception of the world.
- View your patients with compassion, regardless of what they have done with their lives.
- Treat each patient as if he or she were your mother (or another beloved relative, if that works better).

- Stand with the patient as the dying process progresses.
- Figuratively and literally hold the patient's hand.

## The Language of Dying

There was a time, in the Middle Ages, when dying was not considered a big deal (Moller, 1996). You knew something irreversible was happening to your body despite ingesting ancient and blessed potions. You made peace with everyone, tied up loose ends, gave away the furniture, and then just stopped breathing. Now we are afraid to use the "D" word and avoid referring to it, even indirectly, in our hellos and goodbyes.

### Using the "D" Word

In the 1930s, there was a notion that labeling a child as a "stutterer" would lead to severe psychological trauma (Van Riper, 1939). Somewhat illogically, it was thought that despite being teased for repeating and blocking, children who stuttered would not perceive themselves as different from other children. We often do the same thing with people who are dying. Family and friends are afraid of using the "D" word, although these people are aware of what is happening to them. When patients corner physicians for an answer regarding how long they have to live, even the most brilliant clinicians stumble as if they were on a first date.

A number of years ago, I volunteered at George Mark Children's House hospice, in San Leandro, California. Although we did not initiate conversations about dying with children, parents knew that if their child asked us, we would not lie. I remember playing with a 7-year-old boy whose health was rapidly deteriorating. We had gotten close since he had entered the House. As it became harder for him to roll balls to me in a game we had designed, he said, "We won't be able to do this anymore, will we?" I asked him why he thought that and he said, "I think I'm getting closer to dying." I put my arms around him and did not say anything.

Most adults know they are dying even when you do not use the word, and so do many children. I have seen 6-year-olds realize it. Younger children may not have a concept of death, but they realize something very different is happening with their bodies. That understanding may not be apparent in their words, but if you are observant, you will see it in their behaviors—a reluctance to do something, the need to be close to an adult, the desire to do something they are familiar with rather than a new activity. Just as dying adults crave stability, so do dying children. There is a misguided notion that pretending someone is not dying will reduce the trauma. "Ignorance is bliss" works only when everything surrounding the person is conforming to the deception. Yes, the realization that one is dying can be a terrifying experience. Unless the accompanying deterioration is extremely rapid, a person eventually will realize it. The moment of knowing one is going to die is shocking, but for many, it is not as traumatic as reviewing their lives after receiving the news. Difficult deaths occur when people cannot tie up the loose ends or do not have sufficient time to do it.

### What to Do

- Determine the institution's/family's position on talking about death.
- If children ask if they are dying, ask them why they think they are.
- If your patient wants to talk about dying, do not change the subject.
- Do not be afraid to use the words "death" and "dying" if your patient has used them.
- Do not use euphemisms such as "passing on" or "passing away," unless your patient uses them first.
- Mourning is not confined to friends and relatives of the deceased. People who are dying mourn the losses they have already experienced and the ones they will undergo. Do not be afraid to talk about it.

## Greetings and Goodbyes

When greeting patients, we often use stock lines such as "How are you?" Once, I actually had a patient answer: "I'm dying." There are better ways of expressing concern, such as "How have you been this week? or "How has your pain been?" Sometimes it is easier to ask about specific behaviors. A hospice nurse I know always starts her visit with "How's it going?"

Leaving poses another linguistic problem. There is a natural tendency to say, "Goodbye, I'll see you next week." But terminally ill patients know there may not be a next week. In some ways, the phrase perpetuates the fiction. A better approach is to express how much the visit meant to you. I often say, "Thanks for allowing me to visit this week. I enjoyed the time we spent together."

### What to Do

- When greeting, focus on specific behaviors, not general health.
- When leaving, express your appreciation for the visit; do not say that you will see the person the following week.

### Learning from Our Patients

Shared expertise has been a theme of this book. It may not be appropriate to consider ourselves the conveyers of knowledge whose role is to make suggestions that we expect clients and patients to unequivocally accept. Their assessment of your advice is seen through the context of dying, something you can only know tangentially. Start with the assumption that disagreement with your recommendations reflects a difference in experience rather than an unreasonable resistance to your advice. Do not be afraid of becoming involved in your clients' lives. If you are willing to accept that they have as much to contribute to you as you have to contribute to them, you will receive some of the greatest lessons on living (Goldberg, 2010).

### Getting Involved

We hear the often-touted belief that professional distance is a necessary attribute (Maslach, 1993). We are warned that getting close with someone will lead to a loss of objectivity or, worse, caring too much. Well-meaning instructors counsel us: "Don't take your cases home with you—that's the quickest way of burning out." I began experiencing the cost of such involvement early in my hospice work, when during my first month, four of the residents whom I became close to died. Fortunately, a presentation was scheduled by a nurse who, for 15 years, had been involved in hospice work. I asked her how she had been able to accept the loss of the thousands she cared for—how was it possible not to get professional burnout. Her answer was illuminating:

Love can take many forms. The love I experience for my patients involves feeling I've done everything I could have to make their death as peaceful as possible. I know everyone I care for will die within 6 months. If I focused on that, I'd go crazy or quit. But when you know you're helping them on a journey, your love is different. So is your sense of loss. Yes, I miss most of the patients I've worked with, but that's minor compared with what I think I gave them.

Caring too much does not result in burnout. Actually, I have found the reverse to be true. I have never left a bedside quite the same person I was when I sat down. Instead of feeling drained, I am invigorated. Compassion is a strange drug. You will find that the more you give, the more you will receive. Often, the gifts come in the form of lessons.

### What to Do

- Understand that you are not there to fix anything. All of your terminally ill patients will die, no matter what you do.
- Burnout does not come from caring too much. It comes from not realizing that your role is to help the transition between life and death.

## The Lessons

Sogyal Rinpoche (1995) noted that the Buddha said that just as an elephant leaves the biggest footprint in the jungle, so does death when it comes to living. When you are in the presence of someone who will soon die, you probably will have your greatest opportunity for learning how to live. I learned the importance of *forgiveness* from an ex-heroin addict whose family took grim pleasure in the fact that he was dying because they blamed him for the death of his son. I also learned the power of *compassion*, watching an elderly angry woman dramatically change her life one month before she died in my arms. I learned the need for *friendship* from the founder of a historic collection of gay erotic art, afraid he would die alone. I learned *selflessness* from a teenager suffering from cystic fibrosis, who was more concerned about the distress he was causing his mother than the pain he experienced with each breath. And I learned *to live in the present* from a woman who, while holding her infant and knowing he would be dead within a few days, thanked friends and family for a surprise Mother's Day party.

These people and others provided profound lessons that grabbed me and said, "Listen, this is important." I was able to recognize the offering of lessons such as these only after I redefined my role from an SLP to a communication counselor. Even though I was not functioning in a professional capacity in hospice, I brought my professional orientation with me (Goldberg, 2005b). Throughout my career, I viewed what I did as "fixing" or "helping." I worked with children and *fixed* a language problem. With adults, I *helped* persons with aphasia regain the ability to retrieve words or stutterers how to use fluency-enhancing strategies. Your development as a person may reflect what you do in therapy. According to Remen (1997) in her book, *Kitchen Table Wisdom: Stories That Heal*, when you *fix*, you assume something is broken. When you *help*, you see the person as weak. With either perception, there is unequal relationship. It is the one-way street we have gone down our entire professional lives. But when you *serve*, you see the person as intrinsically whole and create a relationship in which both of you grow. The focus shifts from inequities to abilities; to what each can teach the other. As a hospice volunteer, I do not try to fix or help. I serve, and in the process I learn how to live from those who are dying (Goldberg, 2011). As communication specialists, you can do the same.

### What to Do

- Regardless of the disease or the severity, view your patients as whole human beings.
- Listen to people who are dying; they have profound insights into living—what to do and what to avoid.

■ If possible, be present at the death of your patient. It is the greatest spiritual event you will ever witness—other than your own death.

## Conclusion

There is a Cherokee saying that "the heart is the first teacher." As threatening as it may be, allow it to open with dying patients. The poet Rainer Maria Rilke said, "our deepest fears are like dragons guarding our deepest treasures" (Mitchell, 1989). Your patients hold the keys to your locked doors.

## References

Emmon, R. A. (2004). The psychology of gratitude: An introduction. In R. A. Emmons & M. E. McCullough (Eds.), *The psychology of gratitude* (pp. 3–16). New York, NY: Oxford University Press.

Goldberg, S. A. (1997). *Clinical skills for speech-language pathologists.* San Diego, CA: Singular.

Goldberg, S. (2002, September). Reinvent yourself: 10 principles of change. *Psychology Today,* pp. 38–44.

Goldberg, S. A. (2003, June). Are we losing our heart? *ASHA Leader.*

Goldberg, S. (2005a, Winter). A life changed: Lessons learned as a hospice volunteer. *SFSU Magazine, 5,* 1.

Goldberg, S. (2005b). *Ready to learn: How to help your preschooler succeed.* New York, NY: Oxford University Press.

Goldberg, S. (2006). Shedding your fears: Bedside etiquette for dying patients. *Topics in Stroke Rehabilitation, 13*(1), 63–67.

Goldberg, S. (2009a, Oct/Nov). The hard work of dying. *Shambhala Magazine.*

Goldberg, S. (2009b, Winter). Learning from our losses. *Living With Loss.*

Goldberg, S. (2010a). *Lessons for the living: Stories of forgiveness, gratitude, and courage at the end of life.* Boston, MA: Shambhala.

Goldberg, S. (2010b). Lessons for the living. In M. Mclead (Ed.), *Best Buddhist writings of 2010.* Boston, MA: Shambhala.

Goldberg, S. A. (2011, November). How can I be a compassionate caregiver? *Buddhadharma.*

Goldberg, S. (2012). *Leaning into sharp points: Practical guidance and nurturing support for caregivers*. San Rafael, CA: New World Library.

Hanh, T. N. (1991). *Peace is every step*. New York, NY: Bantam Books.

Hanh, T. N. (2000). *The path of emancipation*. Berkeley, CA: Parallax Press.

Kapleau, P. (1989). *The zen of living and dying*. Boston, MA: Shambhala.

Korzybski A. (1958). *Science and sanity*. Lakeville, CT: The International Non-Aristotelian Library.

Krishnamurti, J. (1994). *Commentaries on living*. Madras, India: Quest Books.

Kübler-Ross, E. (1997). *On death and dying*. New York, NY: Scribner.

Maslach, C. (1993). Burnout: A multidimensional perspective. In W. B. Scheaufel, C. Maslach, & T. Marek (Eds.), *Professional burnout: Recent developments in theory and research* (pp. 19–32). New York, NY: CRC Publishers.

Mitchell, S. (Trans.). (1989). *The selected poetry of Rainer Maria Rilke*. New York, NY: Vintage Press.

Moller, D. W. (1996). *Confronting death*. New York, NY: Oxford University Press.

Remen, R. (1997). *Kitchen table wisdom: Stories that heal*. New York, NY: Riverhead.

Rinpoche, P. (1994). *The words of my perfect teacher*. Boston, MA: Shambhala.

Rinpoche, S. (1993). *Tibetan wisdom for living and dying* [Audiotape]. New York, NY: Rigpa Foundation.

Rinpoche, S. (1994). *The Tibetan book of living and dying*. New York, NY: HarperSanFrancisco.

Rinpoche, S. (1995). *Glimpse after glimpse*. New York, NY: HarperSan-Francisco.

Van Riper, C. (1939). *Speech correction: Principles and methods*. New York, NY: Prentice-Hall.

Weber, M. (1946). *Essays in sociology*. New York, NY: Oxford University Press.

# INDEX

**Note:** Page numbers in **bold** reference non-text material.